THE HANDBOOK OF
MEDITERRANEAN
DIET

A Nutrition Book with the Healthiest & Tastiest Recipes Backed by Science

Dr. Theo Christodoulakis, NMD H (ASCP)

ISBN: 978-0-9988-1651-7 (sc)
ISBN: 978-0-9988-1652-4 (hc)
ISBN: 978-0-9988-1653-1 (e)

Library of Congress Control Number: 2017917728

Rev. date: 11/22/2017

Contents

About the Author vii

Famous Quotes ix

Opening Dialogue.. 1

Greek, Italian, French, or Spanish? 2

The Mediterranean Diet 4

Health and Analyzing the Mediterranean Diet........................... 6

Sexual Health and Mediterranean Diet 10

TRADITIONAL vs MODERN Mediterranean Diet 11

Mediterranean Diet is a food culture.. 13

Table Summary of the Mediterranean Diet Foods.................... 15

Diet Principles of the Mediterranean Diet 16

Principles of the Mediterranean Diet explained....................... 17

The Traditional Mediterranean Diet Pyramid 25

Food Categories..26

The Cooking Style of the Mediterranean Diet...........................38

Example of a weekly Mediterranean menu 40

Therapeutic benefits of ingredients found in Med-Diet 43

    Cinnamon (Cassia Cinnamon) 45

    CLOVE (Syzygium aromaticum) 47

    Garlic (Allium sativum)...52

    Oregano (Origanum vulgare) 54

    Sweet Basil (Ocimum basilicum) 56

    MINT...58

    Parsley (Petroselinum crispum) 59

    Bay Leaf (Laurus nobilis)...61

    Sage (Salvia officinalis) 63

    Roman Chamomile (Chamaemelum nobile) 65

    Olive Oil (Olea europaea)...67

    Lemon (Citrus limonum)..70

Tomato (Solanum lycopersicum) 72

Onion Allium cepa 73

English Walnut (Juglans regia) 75

Almond (Prunus amygdalus) 77

Coffee (Coffea arabica, C. robusta) 79

Honey (Apis mellifera) 82

Mastic (Pistacia lentiscus) 84

Wine 86

Mediterranean Diet, also known as: The Greek Diet.............88

Recipes 93

Stuffed zucchini with lemon egg sauce (Avgolemeno)................94

Stuffed zucchini flowers...96

Zucchini Fritters 98

Spinach Pie (Spanakopita) 100

Peas and dill (Arakas)...103

Stuffed grape leaves (dolmadakia)...104

Egg and lemon chicken soup with rice (Avgolemono soupa)...106

Lentil soup (Fakes)..107

Santorini's Fava (Yellow split pea puree) 108

Fish soup (Kakavia)...110

Beef soup with ribs and Bone Marrow....................................112

Giant Beans (Fasolada)..113

Yogurt and cucumber sauce (Tzatziki)....................................114

Skordalia (potato-garlic spread)..115

Baked fish..116

Meat balls in sauce (souzoukakia) 117

Eggplant & Beef (Moussaka)...118

Braised beef and onion stew (Stifado) 121

Stuffed cabbage leaves (lahano dolmathes) 122

Chicken a la Ferrugia 124

Spinach with rice (as a side dish with the chicken
    recipe above)..125

Blanquette de Veau 126

String Beans in tomato sauce.. 128

Braised Artichokes 129

Braised okra (Mbamies Yahni).. 130

Lamb Stew 131

Eggplant stew.. 132

Beetroot salad 133

Dandelion Greens / Radikia 134

Greek Salad.. 135

Baklava 136

Greek Coffee 138

Glossary.. 139

About the Author

A Physician, an Educator and an Author

www.OneGoodDoctor.com

Dr. Theo Christodoulakis NMD, H (ASCP) is a licensed and practicing physician in the state of Arizona, USA. Dr. Theo in addition to his medical license from the great and sunny state of Arizona, also holds a DEA (Drug Enforcement Agency) license and is credentialed with several insurance companies as a specialist.

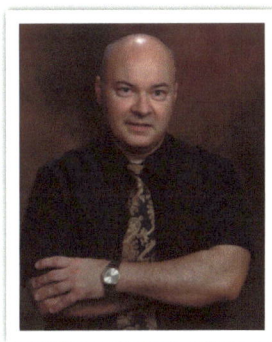

In addition to his Doctorate in Naturopathic Medicine from Southwest College of Naturopathic Medicine, Dr. Theo holds a Bachelor of Science in Biology, and a Bachelor of Science in Mathematics. Dr. Theo is certified in Hematology Technology by UMDNJ (University of Medicine & Dentistry of New Jersey) and is nationally certified by ASCP (American Society of Clinical Pathologists).

Dr. Theo is a teaching adjunct faculty member at the local naturopathic medical school, he is an internationally known speaker on integrative medicine and the use of Bio-identical Hormone Replacement Therapies. He was invited to speak at the American Academy of Anti-Aging Medicine Conference (A4M) in Thailand in 2013, to educate other physicians on his medical approach to Bio-Identical-Hormone-Replacement-Therapy (BHRT). Dr. Theo has given many wellness community lectures to several large and well-known organizations throughout the state of Arizona.

Dr. Theo has his private practice in Chandler Arizona, practicing good Integrative Medicine (IM) with a focus on Natural Bio-Identical Hormones (BHRT) and Food Sensitivities.

<u>His integrative medical approach toward his patients, is:</u>
Quality----personalization---- knowledge--
--common sense----compassion

Dr. Theo Christodoulakis has over 20 years' experience working in various laboratories and hospitals throughout the country, with more than 10 years in primary care, pain management and hormone replacement therapies. Dr. Theo is a second-generation physician.

Famous Quotes

"Let food be thy medicine and medicine be thy food"

Hippocrates, father of medicine c. 460 BC– c. 370 BC

"Illnesses do not come upon us out of the blue. They are developed from small daily sins against Nature. When enough sins have accumulated, illnesses will suddenly appear"

Hippocrates, father of medicine c. 460 – c. 370 BC

Good Food = Good Mood

Unknown

"One bite and all is forgiven."

Unknown

Φάε λάδι και έλα βράδυ. "Eat olive oil and come in the evening." (referring to the aphrodisiac qualities of olive oil; you will enjoy a night of passion)

Unknown, Greek idiom

"The only thing I like better than talking about Food is eating food"

John Walters

"Raw vegetables are for Goats; nice vegetable dishes are for people"

Dr. Theo

Food is multidimensional, it has looks, smells, textures, taste, quality ingredients, a story to tell and can be enjoyed if you know the cook and have a lovely face to look at while you eat.

Dr. Theo

The History of Medicine

2000 BC: Here eat this root

1000 AD: This root is heathen, say this prayer

1850 AD: That prayer is superstition, drink this potion

1920 AD: That potion is snake oil, swallow this pill

1985 AD: This pill is ineffective, take this antibiotic

2000 AD: This antibiotic is artificial, eat this root

The stages of medical acceptance

Stage 1: Don't be stupid, it will never work

Stage 2: Try it, it might work

Stage 3: It's so simple, even a baby could have figured that out

Opening Dialogue

We always hear about the health benefits of a Mediterranean Diet, but do you really know what Mediterranean foods to cook or eat? When I was in medical school in the USA, I always heard about the benefits of the Mediterranean Diet. It was due to my ethnic background that I always have known what Mediterranean cuisine is, and I felt fortunate to have experienced this cultural culinary upbringing. I eventually realized that even though my teachers, my colleagues and the patients knew the healthy benefits of a Mediterranean Diet, they really did not know the cuisine, the actual foods and the dishes. Most people know that olive oil, walnuts, vegetables and fruit are part of the healthy Mediterranean Diet, but very few know how to eat those foods. People do not eat walnuts or drink olive oil for dinner. The wonderful and healthy ingredients are combined into recipes to create mouthwatering and flavorful dishes that nourish the body and soul.

This handbook has the guidelines of the food culture, the ingredients, the top healthiest dishes, and some of the science behind the celebrated Mediterranean Diet.

This is a book dedicated to my love of healthy and flavorsome food, integrative medicine, my parents' upbringing, my wife's patience and to my son. A special thanks to Michelle Epifano-Gidosh for the final proofreading.

Diet, Nutrition, Med-Diet

The word "diet," even though it is associated with weight loss, actually means nutrition. It comes from the Greek word "διατροφή" (diatrophy), which means "nutrition." In this publication, diet refers to nutrition. The Mediterranean diet is sometimes abbreviated as Med-Diet.

Greek, Italian, French, or Spanish?

"Mediterranean" means "middle earth." Several countries surround the region of the Mediterranean Sea: Spain, France, Italy, Greece, modern day Turkey, Israel and North Africa. The Mediterranean region, due to its ideal location and mild weather, promoted an ideal environment for the development of some great civilizations. The exchange of their knowledge and cultures between those countries, which promoted educational advancement, gentility and refinement, also cultivated their cuisine.

Italian Influences: Italian culture is similar to Greek culture but incorporates higher amounts of starches than Greek cuisine. Italians adopted noodles from the Chinese that gave them a whole different level of refinement in their cuisine. Italian cuisine incorporates an abundant use of olive oil, garlic, herbs, wine, coffee, seafood, vegetables, fruit, minimally processed home-cooked food and family time spent eating.

French and Spanish Influences: These cultures incorporate the abundant use of seafood, olive oil, vegetables and the moderate consumption of wine and coffee.

Greek Influences: The Mediterranean diet originally observed the dietary patterns of Greece, Italy, France and Spain, but now it is understood that the Mediterranean diet is mostly associated with the traditional Greek diet. This is perhaps due to the Greek culture, which has a more archaic and isolated development from the other countries mentioned previously. Greek cuisine is more primitive and natural than that of the progressive Renaissance countries. That development, coupled with a civilized environment, created a distinct, idealistic diet with some of the tastiest dishes in the world. Today's traditional Mediterranean diet is seen in Greece and mostly in Crete, an island at the southern part of Greece.

An interesting point is that Greece of today is vastly different from Greece of 2000 years ago, when Greek civilization had surrounded the area around the Mediterranean Sea, spreading its cultural influence over the area. Greek civilization influenced the Roman civilization where, in turn, it took over and surrounded the Mediterranean Sea region.

The Mediterranean Diet

The Mediterranean diet is one of the oldest nutritional patterns and it has existed for about 2000 years. The term "Mediterranean diet" was conceived in the 1940s by observing the reduced incidents of cardiovascular and chronic diseases in the countries surrounded by the Mediterranean Sea, despite the fact, that people there consume an increased amount of fat and animal proteins. The "French paradox" refers to the epidemiological observation in the 1980s, where the French suffer a relatively low incidence of coronary heart disease, despite having a diet relatively rich in saturated fats, a contributing factor for coronary heart disease. (https://www.ncbi.nlm.nih.gov/pmc/articles/PMC1768013/).

It was not until the 1990s, that the Mediterranean diet started to gain acceptance by the medical community as the diet of choice to prevent and reduce cardiovascular disease. By the turn of this century, the Mediterranean diet was also seen as an anti-inflammatory diet used in combating chronic diseases. The Mediterranean diet is mentioned in the 2015–2020 Dietary Guidelines (The Office of Disease Prevention and Health Promotion, www.health.gov) as an example of an eating pattern that promotes good health, a healthy body weight, and disease prevention throughout one's lifespan. The main aspects of this nutritional arrangement include proportionally high consumptions of olive oil, legumes, unrefined grains, fruit, vegetables, and moderate to high consumptions of seafood. It also suggests mild to moderate consumptions of red meat, cheese, and yogurt.

An unhealthy diet is one of the primary factors that contribute to the rise of inflammatory and autoimmune diseases in the populations of both developed and developing countries. These diseases are also referred to as "Chronic Diseases." Chronic diseases such as heart disease, stroke, cancer, type 2 diabetes, obesity, and arthritis are among the most common ones that are preventable. "Chronic diseases are due to unhealthy risk behaviors such as lack of exercise or physical activity, poor nutrition and tobacco use" (CDC.gov.). "Chronic diseases generally cannot be prevented by vaccines or cured by medication, nor do they just disappear" (Medicinenet.com).

Many chronic diseases are due to abnormal inflammation and abnormal responses of the immune system. The Mediterranean diet has been associated with a reduced incidence of certain pathologies related to chronic inflammation and immune system dysregulation. Examples of some of these chronic diseases that may be helped by the Mediterranean diet are several types of arthritis, cardiovascular disease, metabolic syndrome, irritable bowel syndrome and even cancer.

Med-Diet has been promoted in medical schools as the nutrition of choice, but very few professionals know the actual foods, ingredients, and dishes involved in one of the healthiest diets in the world. Beyond studies and research, physicians and nutritionists need to know the Med-Diet and how to explain this way of healthy eating. I often hear in seminars the main ingredients of the Mediterranean diet touted for their benefits, but I quickly realize many people, including physicians, do not know the actual and individual dishes. Many physicians and researchers say, "Eat walnuts, olive oil, vegetables, and fruits". In reality, no one eats walnuts, olive oil, and salad for dinner. Real Mediterranean people eat lentil soup, stuffed zucchini, grape leaves, fava, kouloures, and baklava. This was my inspiration for writing this publication. It is a short course on nutrition in the Mediterranean diet with recipes physicians can pass onto their patients and friends.

Health and Analyzing the Mediterranean Diet

When observing and analyzing all the Mediterranean countries, we see some common characteristics in the healthy Mediterranean diet. These countries and cultures share a mild weather, live close to the sea and have a relaxed attitude toward life. These cultures also share the abundant consumption of seafood, olive oil, vegetables, fruit, grains, moderate use of wine and coffee, incorporation of herbs and spices with the food, moderate daily activity and family eating. The moderate consumption of flour products in these cultures is whole-grain-based, minimally processed foods that provide high amounts of fiber, and innate vitamins and minerals. The typical Mediterranean Diet is natural and simple and without the use of preservatives or chemicals.

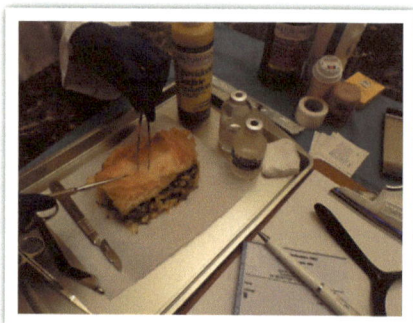

The positive health effects of the Mediterranean diet are undeniable, and many epidemiological studies support the benefits. For example, its high intake of dietary polyphenol reduces the risks for neurodegenerative diseases, heart disease, diabetes, obesity, metabolic syndrome, cancer, cognitive dysfunction, Parkinson's disease, Alzheimer's disease, breast cancer and even early death.

OLIVE OIL is the main health-promoting component of the diet, but other dietary factors are also noted. Other contributing factors to health include the use of unprocessed, non-synthetic foods like the inclusion of fruit, vegetables, whole grains, legumes, nuts, and seeds.

These foods are high in polyphenols, vitamins, minerals and fiber that provide anti-inflammatory and blood sugar–regulating actions needed for a healthy body. The abundant use of olive oil and butter provides fat for growth, development and cell communication through essential fatty acids. Fat consumption is important for the proper function of brain and nerves, forming steroid hormones and transporting nutrients through cell membranes.

SEAFOOD provides important nutrients and minerals important in thyroid function such as zinc, selenium, and iodine. In addition, seafood provides a significant amount of EPA (Eicosapentaenoic acid) and DHA (Docosahexaenoic acid), important in combating inflammation and helping with cognitive function. EPA and DHA help lower inflammatory cytokines such as IL-6 and IL-1β, associated with neurodegenerative and autoimmune diseases.

The use of **PROTEINS** found in legumes, cheese, seafood, and red meat helps facilitate chemical reactions that break down protein to amino acids and help transport molecules throughout our bodies to build muscles and enzymes and they also perform many other important functions within the body.

CARBOHYDRATES in grains are used for immediate energy, whereas the fiber, inside the carbohydrates is used to slow the body's breakdown of carbohydrates and the absorption of sugar, thus helping with blood sugar control and preventing surges and dips of energy. Blood glucose swings are dangerous to the health, because it is linked with oxidative stress that can cause any number of health issues. In addition, Hyperglycemia is associated with the production of AGED (advanced Glycation End Products) that are associated with increased vascular permeability and arterial stiffness, oxidizing LDL and pro-inflammation by inducing the secretion of a variety of cytokines. The simple habit of eating high fiber carbohydrates (instead of simple carbohydrates) can prevent and even treat a variety of chronic diseases associated with abnormal pro-inflammation.

VITAMINS AND MINERALS that are found in vegetables are used in a multitude of reactions and act as the precursors, cofactors needed for thousands of chemical reactions used by the body to build and maintain homeostasis. Several vitamins have endocrine-like actions, involved with coagulation and mediate transcription in bone tissue. (*Curr Opin Investig Drugs. 2006 Oct;7(10):912-5. Vitamins: not just for enzymes. Bolander FF1) - (J Drugs Dermatol. 2007 Aug;6(8):782-7.Vitamins and minerals: their role in nail health and disease. Scheinfeld N1, Dahdah MJ, Scher R), (Clin Dermatol. 2010 Jul-Aug;28(4):420-5. doi: 10.1016/j. clindermatol.2010.03.037. Nutrition and nail disease. Cashman MW1, Sloan SB.)*

WATER has many functions such as enabling hydrolysis that participates in a cell's biochemical reactions, nutrient transport, waste removal, protection of sensitive tissues and temperature regulation.

SALT is not avoided in Med-Diet and has fundamental benefits. In warm weather and in active lifestyles, salt is essential for sustaining hydration levels in the body, maintaining electrolyte balance is crucial for good health, maintaining blood pressure, regulating insulin, and helping to regulate the amount of fluid around and inside the cells. A Mediterranean diet might have just proven that it could be the correct balance of nutrients most human bodies need.

NATURAL, SIMPLE AND ORGANIC describes the ingredients used. The ingredients used in the traditional Mediterranean Diet are picked from the local farm stands or people's own backyards. Many dishes are seasonal and use ingredients like greens (horta) and are often self-picked. The ingredients and herbs are cooked together in a simple and slow way, which helps infuse the flavors. There are no genetically modified foods or pesticides used in the traditional Greek diet.

HOME-COOKED meals is a fundamental concept in a traditional Med-Diet. Food preparation is time consuming, but the results are monumental for health and taste buds alike. A typical Greek dish can take two to three hours to cook. For that reason, it is common to see the housewives engaged in the kitchen for most of the day. In Mediterranean cultures, the matriarch is referred to as the "supporting column of the house," which signifies the importance of the person cooking and taking care of family members. Without the supporting column of the housewife, the home will fall.

Unfortunately, home cooking is quickly becoming a disappearing art in the modern western world, and one of the consequences is health deterioration in the modern lifestyle.

Preparing meals, as we see in the traditional Mediterranean culture is a family bonding ritual. Cooking for loved ones benefits the practitioner, by unwinding and concentrating on the art of healing, through food preparation for their family and friends. The person receiving and accepting the meal are also an unconscious action of approval and consent of the care the matriarch displays. The act of cooking and receiving home-cooked meals is a cultural tradition that have made people civilized and content.

Sexual Health and Mediterranean Diet

Sexual dysfunction due to organic causes is more likely to occur in people suffering from health conditions such as circulatory disorders, coronary heart disease, diabetes, degenerative conditions, neurological and hormonal disorders.

Med-Diet is long recognized and accepted in improving cardiovascular function, increasing blood flow to vessels and organs, improving diabetes and metabolic syndrome and all conditions associated with a poor and unhealthy sexual function in individuals. Adherence to a Mediterranean diet is associated with reduced risks of having high cholesterol and lipids, hypertension, diabetes, metabolic syndrome and obesity, all risk factors for sexual dysfunction.

Several studies have looked at the beneficial effects of the Mediterranean Diet on sexual dysfunction and found that "among persons with diabetes and metabolic syndrome, a Mediterranean diet reduced the deterioration of sexual function over time in both sexes" and that "Med-Diet might be effective in ameliorating sexual function in women and men with metabolic syndrome and cardiovascular disease." The adoption of healthy lifestyles can reduce the prevalence of obesity and the metabolic syndrome, and hopefully the burden of sexual dysfunction.

In addition, Mediterranean cuisine is full of Aphrodisiac foods such as olive oil, almonds, eggs, walnuts, seeds, clove, cinnamon, parsley, honey, royal jelly and a good amount of healthy fats important for hormone synthesis, and brain and nerve functions … So, eat up!

TRADITIONAL vs MODERN
Mediterranean Diet

The Mediterranean diet, also known as the Greek Diet, is rich in heart-healthy fiber and nutrients which includes omega-3 and 9 fatty acids and antioxidants. The diet generally includes: fruits, vegetables and unsaturated fats, particularly olive oil. (Natural Therapeutics)

The traditional Mediterranean diet has changed over the last 50 years and has turned into the "Modern" Diet which does not have the same health benefits as the traditional. The modern Mediterranean diet has started using an enormous amount of highly processed flour products and a lot of breads and spaghetti. Today's flour is highly processed and devoid of the nutrients that were embodied in the traditional diet before processing, additives and preservatives make them unhealthy. The old heavy and whole grain breads is slowly being replaced with its cheaper and lower quality, "fluffy" substitutes. Some cheaper flours are GM (genetically modified) which has possibly contributed in some problematic health conditions like diabetes, arthritis and cancer, which were rare before. The western influence of fast food has permeated into the modern culture and brought along convenient and cheaper foods. Unfortunately, it has also brought diseases of "affluence". *Diseases of affluence are the selected conditions that are a result of increased wealth, food over-consumption and reduced physical activity in a society.*

Prior to 1980 in Greece, there were no fast food restaurants, the family ate home-cooked foods together, at home, and foods were less processed.

This publication is explaining the Traditional Med-Diet. The sad observation is that the new generation of young people, do not adhere to the Mediterranean Diet pattern, even though they live in the lands characterized by the tradition and culture of healthy nutrition, where initially it was discovered.

Mediterranean Diet is a food culture

Med-Diet is the use of healthy and wholesome ingredients in addition to a traditional culture of home cooking and eating with the family.

Healthy food + healthy living = Mediterranean Diet

One thing that is always overlooked in the Mediterranean cuisine is the culture. The culture is important because it teaches us "how" to eat those healthy foods. If we only consider the healthy ingredients of Med-Diet without considering how and when to eat, we will be missing on the complete benefits of this Diet. Some foods in the traditional Med-Diet might appear to be not so healthy, but the habits, cooking styles and outside factors like family time eating, turn it into a healthy diet. A perfect example is the eating of baklava, a very high calorie dessert. Even though baklava is full of sugar, it does not have synthetic and highly processed ingredients. The sweetener used is honey, and the filling is made of natural walnuts full of nutrients and oils. In addition, a piece of baklava is enjoyed as a splurge on special occasions and eaten at a slow pace, while enjoying friends and family. Baklava is not usually eaten right after the meal, but rather as a day break snack along with coffee or tea.

Mediterranean culture is relaxed and laid back. Eating food is a social behavior to share time with family and friends. We often see people taking evening or late-night coffee or tea breaks with friends that last 1-2 hours. Eating dinner can take 1-3 hours to complete, because it is common to socialize while eating. When people go to a tavern to eat dinner, it is usually a social function that involves the entire evening. It is often said that the tavern customer "owns" the table for the whole night. Customers are not rushed to finish their food which is in contrast to the American lifestyle.

It is this type of mentality, behavior and culture, has given the reputation of the Mediterranean people as "less productive." The real question is, are the Mediterranean people less productive or more content with life? That question will be perhaps, addressed in a future publication.

Table Summary of the Mediterranean Diet Foods

Table Summary of the Mediterranean Diet Foods:

Abundant consumption of seafood, vegetables,
fruit, legumes, olive oil, seeds and nuts.

Mild to moderate consumption of unrefined
grains, yogurt, cheese, wine and coffee

Mild consumption of red meat, chicken and wild game meat

Mild consumption of honey, sugar, butter

Preservatives and synthetic ingredients are extremely rare

Diet Principles of the Mediterranean Diet

Principles of the Mediterranean Diet:

Moderation and a variety of foods

Eat at 80% full, most of the time

Splurge on the things you like on special occasions only

Eat with friends and family

Eating dinner with friends and family on
the week-end takes 2-3 hours

Taking it easy most of the time

Avoid medications and hospitals as much as possible

When feeling sick drink an herbal tea
like sage or chamomile tea

Walk a lot and sweat often

Breakfast is minimal

Lunch is substantial

Dinner is very light on the weekdays and
heavy but balanced on the weekends

There are no candies or cereals

Comfort foods are spinach-pie and grilled
octopus not macaroni and cheese

Principles of the Mediterranean Diet explained

Moderation and a variety of foods:

Moderation is the avoidance of extremes and excess. Excess of any type of food is linked to diseases of affluence. Moderation teaches self-restrain and more enjoyment of life. Moderation or Homeostasis is a basic function or all living things that lead to a normalization of body functions. Extreme eating of one food or many foods, leads to higher spikes and drops of blood sugar, called dysglycemia, and eventually can lead to metabolic syndrome. The principle of eating in moderation perhaps was developed out of necessity that poor cultures, such as the Greeks and Italians 50 years ago, ate little with cheap and primary ingredients such as beans, lentils and peas. Fish was more available so it was eaten 2-4 times a week whereas red meat was a luxury and it was eaten 1-2 times a week. That moderation contributed to their healthy (Mediterranean) diet.

Moderation was taught in Ancient Greece, Christianity, Buddhism, Taoism and other ancient cultures. There is also an ancient Greek proverb "παν μέτρον άριστον" stating "everything in moderation leads to excellence".

Variety:

Eating one food over and over again, can lead to allergies and nutritional deficiencies. No single food can provide all of the nutrients in the amounts that the body needs. Eating a variety of healthy foods becomes the "safety net" in providing the body the numerous nutrients it needs for normal functioning. In medicine, allergies develop due to over-exposure of an ingredient that induces an abnormal response of the immune system, called hypersensitization.

In Mediterranean cultures, we see a variety of food dishes on small plates. That variety is not the same as appetizers. Appetizers are taken before a meal or the main course of a meal to stimulate one's appetite.

The "variety dishes" in Spain, France, Italy and Greece are different from the "appetizers" in that, *it is the meal.* In Greece the variety dishes are called "mezedes" or "poikilia", in Spain "tapas", in Italy called "cicchetti", in France "hors d'oeuvr" and even the Chinese have "Dim Sum". The serving of those variety dishes is designed to encourage conversation and not focus on the food so much. Most of those dishes are accompanied with wine. The culture of eating a variety of food while socializing allows a greater intake of nutrients, while promoting a longer digestion time during socializing.

Eat at 80% full, most of the times:

The concept of eating less is a well-established method of achieving health that is documented even at the time of Hippocrates 380 BC. Nowadays, much medical research shows that eating less and even fasting overnight can balance and stimulate your growth hormone and give your body time to recover. Growth hormone (GH) is often called the anti-aging hormone due to its beneficial effects on cell growth, increased strength and metabolism. Growth hormone (GH) is stimulated during exercise, night sleeping, and food restriction. In the near future, scientist will agree that this happens with other hormones. The Greek word of λιτοδίαιτος, promotes the idea of undereating but does not have an exact translation in English. Λιτοδίαιτος is a synonym for an eater that is "frugal, restrained, and under-eats or does not self-indulge".

Splurge on the things you like on special occasions only:

What is living without enjoyment? Having fun is fundamental in good health and happiness. Overeating is seen in the Med-Diet culture, on holidays, birthdays, weddings and on special occasions. Special occasions are just that, special, meaning once in a while. In western countries and especially in USA, special occasions and over-indulgence is done almost every day which makes the "special" occasion less special, insignificant and unworthy. Traditional Greek living was minimal, with the occasional "splurging" during special situations.

Eat with friends and family:

In Mediterranean culture, the coming together to exchange knowledge, memories and passion was done by sharing food and enjoying a meal with friends, family members and coworkers.

These cultures enjoy and deem important the interaction with other people. The meal sharing and socializing is seen during dinner which can take anywhere from an hour to 3 hours. The talking and sharing of life experiences allows a person time to relax, enjoy food, chew slower and promotes a longer digestion time. Eating with others puts a restrain in overeating. Sharing a meal is also sharing the calories. Fast food restaurants were not seen in the Traditional Greek Diet, before 1980.

Taking it easy most of the time:

Mediterranean cultures sometimes are seen as less "productive," in comparison with other Northern European and American cultures. The reality is that the good weather and good food of the Mediterranean region promotes a less "hurry up" culture, less stress that leads to slower eating, more time with family and friends, and more enjoyment and appreciation of life. Stress is a state of "threatened homeostasis" that negatively affects the regulation of hormones, immune function and increases free radicals. High stress produces an increased amount of adrenaline and cortisol among other hormones, which contributes to a constant alarmed and inflammatory state, leading to hormone and immune dysregulation and eventual exhaustion as seen in Adrenal Fatigue. A slower pace of life contributes to proper digestion, proper sleep pattern, better mood and blood sugar regulation and fewer accidents. Stress is a contributing factor, and provides an increased risk, in developing cardiovascular diseases, metabolic syndrome, depression, weight gain and a range of chronic diseases. Stress can be managed by being social, happy, a change of situation perception, and with the mild consumption of wine as seen in Mediterranean cultures.

Wine 1-3 times a week.

Wine is the often-overlooked contributor of the Mediterranean Diet benefits. Wine has high amounts of resveratrol, polyphenols and anti-oxidants that are linked to the fight against free radicals, oxidative stress and help with improving health. Oxidative stress is the attack on biological cells that create damage. Oxidative stress is linked as a contributory factor to many diseases such as atherosclerosis, Parkinson's disease, Alzheimer's, cataracts and other chronic diseases.

An additional benefit of wine is, that it is a natural anxiolytic (reduces stress) with much less side effects of pharmaceuticals like alprazolam or diazepam. People in the Mediterranean region use wine as a social "medicine" to help them relax and forget their worries. The consumption of wine or other alcoholic drinks in the med-diet is mild to moderate, and you rarely see a problem with abuse of alcohol as seen in some western societies.

Avoid unnecessary medications and hospital visits as much as possible

In the traditional Greek culture, medications are infrequently used and it is common to have an 80-year-old person without taking any medications at all. While modern western countries often rely on anti-anxiety and anti-depression medications like Xanax and Zoloft, Greeks have incorporated wine and ouzo as a way to forget their problems, at least temporarily. That temporary behavior "shuts off" the "alarm response," and allows the brain and body to downregulate the hyper adrenal response which can lead to several hormonal disorders of over production, and eventual underproduction of the adrenal glands. Greeks, instead of going to psychiatrists, they will spend more time with friends and family.

Herbal drinks are often used for minor health problems. Some of the most common herbal teas are Sage and Chamomile. The famous anti-viral mountain tea Sage and the digestive relaxant Chamomile is found in almost every person's kitchen cabinet. The inclusion of abundant herbs in the Mediterranean cuisine has definitely contributed to the health benefits and reduction of reliance on pharmaceutical medications. Other common herbs used in Med-Diet with medicinal properties are Bay leaves, Oregano, Cloves and Cinnamon.

Pharmaceuticals have a high degree of side effects, complications and interactions. In addition, unnecessary procedures, medications and medical mistakes are causes of harmful effects of 20th century medicine. "Iatrogenic diseases", a less known medical term, is one of the leading causes of death and injury in the Western world.

Iatrogenic translates into "made due to medicine" (procedures and pharmaceuticals) that causes diseases (damages). Although, it is easy to blame physicians and medical institutions for this problem, in reality, the patients share an equal responsibility of this "iatrogenic disease" by "demanding" miracle pills and magical surgeries. People in western civilizations enjoy a high degree of medical advances, but that has caused an over reliance and "perceived need" to pharmaceutical medications for even the simplest health concerns.

In contrast to the USA population, where it demands more medical procedures and pharmaceuticals, Mediterranean cultures like the Greeks, use herbal drinks and natural remedies to resolve simple ailments. It is unusual to see older people in Greece on continuous and chronic medications, in contrast to older people in the USA, where they might be on several medications on a regular basis. In Greece, the use of the mountain tea or sage is used often to help when feeling sick such as the common cold or the flu. Chamomile, another popular herbal drink, is a good calmative and carminative remedy that is used to promote restful sleeping and reduce digestive issues.

Iatrogenic causes of death or injury can be due to side effects, complications, medical or patient errors, negligence, interactions, unnecessary treatments for profit, or anxiety due to a procedure.

Walk a lot and sweat often:

Physical activity is often seen in Mediterranean cultures, and the degree depends on the location. People on the Greek isles where the most health benefits are seen, have the highest degree of activity (Ikaria study). The Ikaria study showed that Med-Diet contributes to longevity where Ikarians were reaching the age of 100 and beyond, a rate 2.5 times that of Americans. The life expectancy in Ikaria exceeded the American average by about a decade. The Ikarian centenarians were also healthier and happier. Ikaria is an island in Greece where it has been called "The island where people forget to die" referring to the high number of centenarians living there. In addition to their diet, their daily activity is definitely a contributing factor to their longevity.

Most people in Greece walk at least an hour a day and sometimes even more. The increased amount of activity leads to increase perspiration and respiration, which helps in the body's detoxification through the skin and the pulmonary system. Increased activity in humans is beneficial with metabolism, muscle tone, bone strengthening and with the reduction of anxiety.

The Ikaria study:
https://www.ncbi.nlm.nih.gov/pmc/articles/PMC3051199/

Breakfast is minimal

The usual breakfast is coffee and a biscotti. Sometimes an egg, a rusk and a piece of cheese can be part of breakfast. A snack will follow 1-2 hours later. The snack might be a cheese pie or a spinach pie with a juice drink. The exact mechanism of the beneficial effects of small breakfast is not fully understood, but it has to do with the totality of the Mediterranean Diet.

Lunch is substantial

The amount of food for lunch is more than the amount of food for dinner. A typical lunch can be stuffed tomatoes, cheese, bread and a drink.

Dinner is light

Dinner is very light on the weekdays and heavy but balanced on the weekends. A light dinner has been observed in the Mediterranean Diet, and it is perhaps the strongest beneficial factor of the food culture. A typical dinner can be tea, a rusk, a piece of cheese, fruit and a yogurt. Once or twice a week people will splurge during dinner, where they will enjoy going to a tavern with friends and family. Alcoholic drinks are enjoyed during dinner on those special outings.

There are no candies or cereals:

There are no artificial and colorful food substitutes in Mediterranean cuisine. We rarely see food coloring added to foods, with the exception of painting Easter eggs. The only preservatives used, are salt, sugar and vinegar, and never un-pronounceable chemicals.

Boxed cereals are never consumed. On occasion, people will have some porridge such as oatmeal or Trahana. *"Trahana"* which is a fermented mixture of whole grains, that is made into a thick soup, with water, stock, or milk. Sometimes yogurt or fermented yogurt is added. In the USA the many varieties of cereals have led to the overconsumption of carbohydrates. 100 years ago, Dr. John Harvey Kellogg, the inspiration of Kellogg's Corn Flakes, was a proponent of a healthy breakfast, but I am sure he did not intend for today's high sugar cereals to be called a "healthy breakfast."

There are no candies or "colorful sugar beans" in Med-Diet. The closest thing to candy, are the chocolate bars (plain or with nuts), cakes, baklava and holiday cookies.

Comfort foods:

When you ask most Americans, what their favorite comfort foods are, you will hear responses of pizza, macaroni and cheese, or French fries (nothing French about it). Most Greek people's comfort foods will be spinach pies, grilled octopus, fava peas or stuffed tomatoes. The reason is, that those foods, even though healthy, actually taste very good. I always say: "eat vegetables because they taste good, not just because there healthy,© a concept which you will never understand, until you have tried some of the tasty recipes included in this book.

The Traditional Mediterranean Diet Pyramid

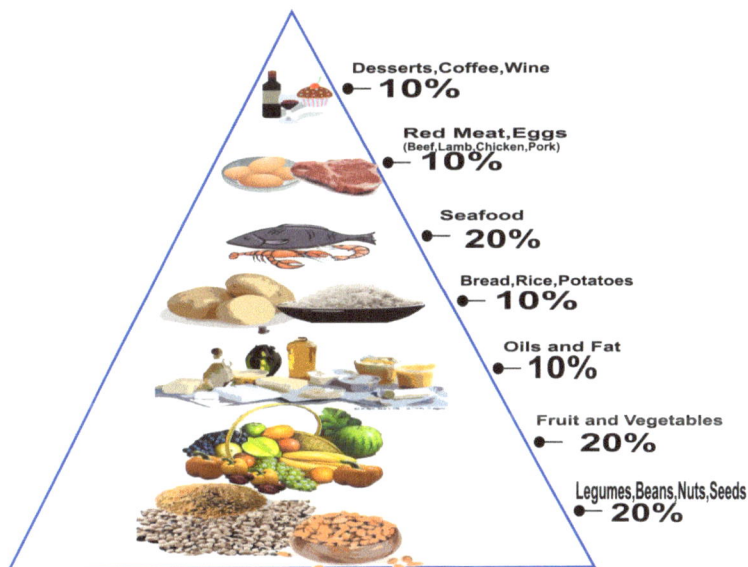

Desserts,Coffee,Wine
10%

Red Meat,Eggs
(Beef,Lamb,Chicken,Pork)
10%

Seafood
20%

Bread,Rice,Potatoes
10%

Oils and Fat
10%

Fruit and Vegetables
20%

Legumes,Beans,Nuts,Seeds
20%

The Foundation:
Simple,Natural,Minimally Processed,Organic,Home-made

The Traditional Mediterranean Diet Pyramid ©
Dr. Theo Christodoulakis
www.OneGoodDoctor.com

Food Categories

Protein:

Seafood is enjoyed more often than red meat. Seafood is eaten 5-7 times a week depending on the area you live in. The most common seafood is white fish, octopus, squid and shrimp. Fish types are sardines, smelt, anchovies, mackerel, bogue, red porgy, sea bass, pandora, dentex and mullet to name few. Almost all kinds of sea creatures are consumed depending on the geographic area. Salmon is not a local fish so it is rarely eaten.

Animal Meat is encouraged but it is only consumed 1-2 times a week. Lamb, goat and beef is more common and chicken coming in as a secondary and more affordable meat. There are some organ meats consumed in small quantities. We often see traditional cultures having nothing go to waste. *(I discourage eating chicken because of the excessive amount of estrogen found inside the meat).*

Eggs are not only eaten for breakfast, but also for lunch or dinner, and can be incorporated into recipes such as in "avgolemono" soup or sauce over stuffed vegetable dishes (zucchini) and meatballs. 2-10 eggs a week is a reasonable amount that a traditional Greek will consume.

Legumes. The "poor man's meat" are the legumes that contain a significant amount of protein at an affordable price that are packed with vitamins, minerals and fiber. There are numerous recipes with lentils, fava peas, and a variety of other beans. Legumes and nuts also have starch and fiber for energy in addition to healthy Omega 3 fats, and B-vitamins.

Spices and herbs:

There are several spices used in the Greek cuisine. The most common spices and herbs used in cooking are garlic, onions, cinnamon, cloves, nutmeg, oregano, basil, mint, salt, and black pepper. Spices have medicinal effects in addition to enhancing flavor benefits.

Starches:

There are side dishes in Greek cuisine that include starches. The most popular dishes are oven lemon potatoes, rice pilaf, spaghetti and of course bread. The bread is similar to Italian style bread, and is used to soak and absorb the oil or the tomato sauce.

Fats and Oil:

Everything is cooked in olive oil. Food is moist and oily and that makes the food taste good and easy to swallow. Olive oil is mostly a monounsaturated oil that has high amounts of antioxidants, and polyphenols that protects against oxidation of blood lipids and has positive effects on cardiovascular health. Olive oil is beneficial when eaten in salads and used in cooking. Olive oil can resist moderate amounts of heat during cooking. Olive oil has a smoke point of around 380 F (193 C). Some other cooking oils" breaks" during the heating process of cooking, causing trans-fats to form, which are linked to cancers and other diseases.

The Smoke point is the temperature at which the oil smokes, indicating that the oil "breaks" causing increased Trans-fatty acids which are proven to be harmful to human health. Other oils that have become fads, such as coconut oils are more resistance in the heating process but have higher amounts of saturated fats, something that most westerners consume plenty of anyway.

Olive oil is a much healthier choice. Olive oil is a fruit juice, produced by the fruit of the olive, and when it is processed it does not need heat or an excessive amount of pressure, therefore, less chances of producing trans-fats during the oil production. Olive oil is consumed in great quantities, and on a daily basis, in the Mediterranean culture. If you consider all of the oil, included in cooking and in salads, a half to a whole (½ -1) cup of olive oil is a realistic amount, that a traditional Greek, Italian or Spaniard person will consume on a daily basis. I often prescribe to my patients to include 1 Tsp. to half a cup of olive oil in their morning smoothie. Olive oil helps with constipation, arthritis, dry skin, cognitive function, decreased libido, cardiovascular benefits, anti-aging and wellness support. Olive oil is an Omega-9 fat and it has anti-inflammatory benefits similar to Omega-3 fats. Omega 3 and Omega-9 have similar benefits to COX-2 inhibitor medications used as an anti-inflammatory, but with fewer side effects. http://themedicalbiochemistrypage.org/omegafats.php

A word of caution: Olive oil has become so valuable and in great demand, that we have started to see adulteration of olive oils by manufactures who are mixing low grade oils such as canola, soybean oil and colza (grapeseed) oil, with coloring and flavorings. Use olive oil from a reputable source.

Vegetables and Vegetarians:

"Raw vegetables are for Goats, whereas nice vegetable dishes are for people,"™ … … … by Dr. Theo.

The majority of vegetable dishes in Greek cuisine are cooked. Cooked vegetables as in baked, sauté, inside soups and even stir fried, they are healthier than raw vegetables. When the vegetables are slightly cooked, the vegetable cell walls break, and the vegetable nutrients are easier to be absorbed and digested by our bodies. Raw vegetables are mostly good as fiber with smaller amounts of nutrient absorption by our bodies.

There is no such thing as "vegetarian" dishes in Greece, but rather vegetable dishes. The difference is, Greek vegetable dishes are made to taste good, and sometimes are cooked with chicken broth or a little bit of meat. There are a group of recipes called "Nistisima" (fasting) or "ladera" (oily) which are the healthiest and most fundamental dishes in Greek cuisine.

Greek Vegetable dishes are the tastiest foods in Greek cuisine, with so many varieties that make life exciting. Try to explore all of them. My favorite vegetable dishes are the "stuffed zucchini flowers", and eggplant dishes such as "papoutsakia", moussaka or eggplant stew.

"Eat vegetables because they taste good, not because you have too," by Dr. Theo.

<u>Fruit:</u>

Fruit is natures' dessert and Greeks enjoy them a lot, especially in the summer. The most popular fruit are grapes, watermelon, figs, apples, oranges and mandarins. Most fruits include vitamins, minerals and fructose that help with digestion.

<u>Grains:</u>

Grains that are minimally processed are consumed with main dishes. Starchy foods like bread, rice and potatoes are eaten as a *"complimentary"* to the main dish. In some western countries grains have become the "main" dish which can lead to overconsumption of carbohydrates.

Some Greek occupations, like farmers and animal herders, perform a lot of manual work and require the consumption of more starches. These people eat dishes like "trahana," a porridge made from minimally processed bulgur wheat. Most modern, commercially made breads, lack the unprocessed and full fiber grains as seen 50 years ago.

Another example of minimally processed grains is "Kritikes Kouloures" or "Kouloures." Kouloures are whole grain hard bagels that are made of barley with the flavor of fennel and are often eaten instead of bread.

Kouloures are high in fiber and many times come with fennel seeds. Kouloures are eaten by slightly softening them with water right before eating, and adding olive oil, oregano and feta cheese. They are a simple and delicious food.

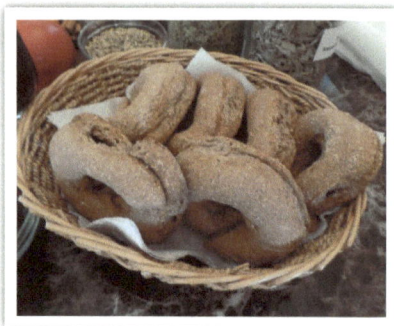

Soups:

Soups are hearty and eaten as a main dish, usually with something on the side, like cheese, bread or a salad. Most common soups are Fakies (lentil soup), Avgolemono (egg-lemon) soup or Kakavia (fish head) soup. Soups are particularly healthy since all the ingredients are retained and infused inside the meal. The soup ingredients are easier to digest since they are softened during cooking. It is common medical knowledge that warm temperature improves digestion, whereas, cold temperature slows digestion. Eating warm foods like soups not only improves digestion, but is also more satisfying and filling.

Refreshments:

Greeks enjoy drinking juice drinks with their meals or alone. Common refreshments are lemonade, orangeade, and a sour-sweet cherry drink called "Visinada". Tart cherry juice is a remedy touted for rheumatism and has anti-inflammatory actions in herbal medicine.

(Crit Rev Food Sci Nutr. 2017 Sep 28:0. doi: 10.1080/10408398.2017.1384918. Tart Cherries and health: Current knowledge and need for a better understanding of the fate of phytochemicals in the human gastrointestinal

tract. Mayta-Apaza AC1, Marasini D1, Carbonero) (J Food Sci. 2012 May;77(5):H105-12. doi: 10.1111/j.1750-3841.2012.02681.x.

Processed tart cherry products--comparative phytochemical content, in vitro antioxidant capacity and in vitro anti-inflammatory activity. Ou B1, Bosak KN, Brickner PR, Iezzoni DG, Seymour EM)

Desserts & Sweets:

Sweets are enjoyed in perhaps larger quantities than they should be, but it is balanced with natural ingredients such as walnuts, honey, and the rest of the healthy Mediterranean lifestyles that are explained throughout this publication. Desserts and sweets are occasionally eaten in special situations. There are no colorful synthetic candies in the traditional Greek cuisine. Common spices used for "sweets" are cinnamon, cloves, nutmeg and occasional sesame and mastiha. Desserts are enjoyed with the company of family and friends during an outing and not in front of the TV, where people forget to stop eating. There is actually a recipe included in this publication, using cups of yogurt and fruit (Yiaourtoglyco) instead of using heavy cream.

Baklava is perhaps the most well-known dessert. Baklava includes ample amounts of honey instead of sugar, and lots of walnuts, and it is eaten as a special treat with friends, a couple of hours away from a meal. There are other sweet pastries that are popular and enjoyed as a snack in between meals with some coffee or tea. Some popular pastries are baklava, kataifi, galactoboureko. There are some cookies that are usually enjoyed during the holidays. Some examples of those cookies are kourambiedes, melomakarouna, and butter cookies. Other popular sweets are yogurt with honey, sesamomelo and "spoon sweets". Sesamomelo is a simple dessert that includes sesame seeds mixed with honey and served on a plate with a spoon on the side. Sesamomelo can also be made into snack bars and are called "pasteli".

Another type of traditional sweets is the "spoon sweet" or "glyco tou koutaliou". Spoon sweets are preserved pieces of fruit with sugar and lemon. These sweets are made of almost any fruit and are sweet, sour and bitter all at the same time. Spoon sweets are also seen in other countries in the Balkans and are a gesture of hospitality in Greece.

Another famous sweet is the mastiha sugar taffy, simply called "mastiha". Mastiha is served on a spoon and rests inside a glass of cold and refreshing water, and it is licked like taffy. This dessert is called "Ypovrihio" which is translated into "submarine" because of its presentation. The main ingredient of this dessert is "Pistacia lentiscus" or mastic which is a therapeutic ingredient traditionally used for the treatment of digestive ailments; such as Helicobacter pylori induced peptic ulcers. Mastica also has many culinary uses.

Cheese:

The main cheese in Greek culture is a fresh goat cheese called Feta. Feta is made of sheep's milk and is considered a fresh cheese with a light, savory and salty flavor. There are other cheeses used such as anthotyri, manouri and some aged cheeses like Kasseri and Graviera. Cheese is eaten on the side of the main dish, and is eaten to add and balance the saltiness of food. Even though Greek food is salty, the Greek culture of daily walking, and the warm weather, which make people sweat, makes salty food a necessity.

Yogurt:

Yogurt is a food produced by the bacterial fermentation of milk referred to as yogurt cultures. The traditional Greek yogurt is made from sheep's milk, it is strained, full fat, tangy, containing a higher protein density than regular yogurt, and has a high amount of bacterial cultures knows as "probiotics." Probiotics are the healthy bacteria that balance the gut flora and are associated with multiple health benefits. Probiotics has become the standard of medicine when patients are on long term antibiotics or have diarrhea. Clinically relevant conditions helped with probiotics are colic, constipation, diarrhea, irritable bowel syndrome, ulcerative colitis, allergies and sensitivities, immune function, infections, stress and even depression. Probiotic bacteria in yogurt can favorably alter the intestinal microflora balance, inhibit the growth of harmful bacteria, promote good digestion, boost immune function, and increase resistance to infections.

Sweet and flavored yogurt is not common in Greece, but the addition of honey, fruit and walnuts is often enjoyed as a special dessert.

Yogurt with honey and walnuts, is a treat that tastes good and it is very healthy. It is simple to prepare and it is a nice ending to a good meal. Greek yogurt is placed on the bottom of the bowl, honey is added on top of the yogurt, and then topped with walnuts. The honey is not mixed with the rest of the ingredients but it is rather scooped and eaten allowing each bite to be different than the other. The taste is sweet, tangy and refreshing.

Nuts and seeds:

Greeks eat a lot of nuts like almonds, walnuts, pumpkin seeds, peanuts, pine nuts, sesame, hazelnuts, chestnuts, and pistachios to name a few. Almost all these nuts are roasted and lightly salted. In the Mediterranean diet, nuts are **not** candied, sugared or honey-roasted. Nuts like peanuts, almonds and walnuts are consumed as snacks in between meals and with alcoholic beverages. Almonds are used as base material in a great variety of desserts. Almonds are considered an aphrodisiac food and recent studies have revealed their benefit in cardiovascular health. Almonds are a symbol of fertility and are often used at weddings as "favors" and gifts to guests.

Nuts are eaten for breakfast with fruit, as a snack with raisins and grapes, and with alcoholic drinks. In addition, there are a large variety of sweets that use nuts as a main ingredient.

Nuts have healthy and essential unsaturated and monounsaturated fats including linoleic acid and essential amino acids in addition to vitamin E, vitamin B2, folate, fiber, and the essential minerals magnesium, phosphorus, potassium, copper, and selenium. Nut consumption is associated with lower mortality from ischemic heart disease, and cardiovascular disease. Eating nuts can lower serum low density lipoprotein (LDL). Nuts also have a very low glycemic index, and are recommended to be included in diets for patients with insulin resistance; such as diabetes and metabolic syndrome.

Coffee:

Greek coffee and an iced coffee called "Frappe" are very common in Greece and are enjoyed in moderation (1-2 cups a day). In Italy they drink espresso and in France Café Noir. The similarities between those countries are that all the coffee preparations are strong (more concentrated) and enjoyed in moderation. Greek coffee is not filtered when it is brewed it has sediment that will not or *should not* be consumed. Coffee is a good herbal drink that helps with constipation, works as a diuretic, increases cognitive function and prevents dementia.

Evidence suggests that long-term consumption of moderate coffee consumption is associated with a lower risk of developing type 2-diabetes, preventing cardiovascular disease and Alzheimer disease.

Drinks and wine

The ancient Greeks were pioneers in yet another science, viticulture, the study of wine production. Many mannerisms and cultural aspects in Greece and Italy were associated with wine that included important religious, social and medicinal purposes. The medicinal use of wine was frequently studied by the Greeks, including Hippocrates the father of medicine, who used wine as a treatment for fevers, analgesic, antiseptic, diuretic, tonic, digestive aid and to ease convalescence. Today wine is well documented in pathology books as beneficial in lowering cholesterol and triglycerides.

There is no significant alcohol abuse in Greece and there is no legal age to start (or stop) drinking. The benefits of wine are well documented when it comes to its moderate and occasional use of 1-2 glasses of red wine consumption. The abuse of alcoholic drinks is also documented, and has the opposite effects that can lead to liver cirrhosis among other health problems. In Mediterranean culture, Alcoholic drinks are used to enjoy someone's company and to relax from everyday stress. Wine drinking is done about 2-3x a week with 2-3 glasses at a time.

There are several different types of wines in Greece. Most wines are made out of grapes and are red, white or rose. Retsina is a wine that has an additional flavor that has the addition of a pine tree resin. Retsina is a strong pungent wine, that has been used for more than 2000 years. The benefits of Retsina have not been researched but many people enjoy that traditional flavor.

There are several alcoholic drinks enjoyed in Greece, but wine is the most popular one. Beer is the second most often consumed alcoholic drink. It is consumed as a refreshing drink during the summer months.

There are other alcoholic drinks such as Tsipouto, Raki, Ouzo, Metaxa and Mastiha.

At special occasions, liquor and liqueur is consumed. Raki or Tsihoudia is a very strong grape based pomace brandy served as an aperitif or digestif. These alcoholic drinks can be bought or are made by people. Ouzo is an anise flavored aperitif drink that is often mixed with water or ice that turns white due to the crystallization of anise with water.

Raki, Tsipouro and Ouzo are very strong alcoholic drinks, and are almost always accompanied with "snacks."

Metaxa drink is an alcoholic drink that is made of brandy, mixed with a Muscat wine and some special flavors. Metaxa drink has been around for about 100 years and has a special distinct flavor.

Wine is an integral part of the Greeks, Italians, French and Spaniards. Drinking wine is a fundamental aspect of the therapeutic effects of the Mediterranean Diet. Wine is a muscle relaxant to help people forget the stress of everyday life. Chronic mild wine consumption is associated with a decreased risk of heart disease, stroke, diabetes mellitus, and early death.

Mild to moderate alcohol use (one to two drinks per day) reduces the risk of coronary heart disease, atherosclerosis, and myocardial infarction (MI), by approximately 30% to 50% when compared with nondrinkers. Heavy alcoholic consumption is associated with liver disease and alcoholism.

Mastica, is another alcoholic drink that is very aromatic and flavorful. Mastica exists as a liquor and liqueur and has the inclusion of Mastic (Pistacia lentiscus), a tree resin found only on one island in the whole world, the island is Chios. Mastic or Mastiha alcoholic drinks have a distinct and an aromatic flavor which should be experienced.

Mastic is also used in baked goods. Mastic, Mastiha or tears of Chios is a resin or a sap obtained from the mastic tree (Pistacia lentiscus) traditionally found on the island of Chios, Greece. The flavor has a refreshing, vanilla and pistachio smell or slightly pine or cedar-like flavor. In Greece, traditional use in foods is for baking, cooking, chewing gums and ice cream. Mastic is used in a "spoon sweet" known as "submarine" (ypovríchio", υποβρύχιο). Trying the flavor of mastiha is a truly unique experience and "a must try" thing to do.

Mastic resin was known since antiquity for its health benefits, and it was first used as the first natural chewing gum. The word "mastication" or chewing has contributed to the name of mastiha or it could be the other way around. It was traded by the Greeks of the island of Chios and it was appreciated as much as "gold" for its many therapeutic and culinary benefits. Several studies have concluded that the use of mastic resin has beneficial actions against Helicobacter pylori, the agent that causes gastritis and stomach ulcers.

https://www.ncbi.nlm.nih.gov/pubmed/19879118,
http://www.mastihashopny.com/files/File/PDF/recipebooklet.pdf

The Cooking Style of the Mediterranean Diet

There are 5 basic cooking methods in cooking Mediterranean style.

1. Baked
2. On the stove top soaked in olive oil
3. Charcoal BBQ cooking
4. Fried
5. Crock pot style.

Charcoal BBQ cooking is the favorite way of enjoying meat when the situation allows. This method drains the excess fat off the meat and provides a well cooked and flavorful meat. The meat is simple seasoned and there are no heavy sauces used. Many taverns and restaurants in Greece cook their meats this way.

Baking in the oven or on the stove top is very healthy because the juices and the nutrients are maintained inside the dish. When cooking on the stove top, the temperature originally reaches the boiling point, and then the food gets simmered at lower temperatures for 45 minutes to up to 2 hours. This technique infuses the spices and herbs with the food, creating therapeutic and flavorful nourishment.

The **crock pot** style of cooking, is usually done outside of the house where the food is prepared in clay pots and then "buried" in the ground with fired charcoals on top. This way of cooking, has a very long preparation time (2-6 hours) and is done at special occasions such as Easter or other important holidays. The end product of this way of cooking, creates a very tender meat, and is a medley of food heaven.

Fried: In Modern Greek cuisine, there are several dishes that are fried in olive oil. Many vegetables like zucchini, eggplant and potatoes are fried due to convenience.

The ingredients are simple, natural, minimally processed and almost always herbs and spices are included. There are no artificial ingredients and preservatives. In most cases local ingredients are used.

Greek food is moist, oily, and full of flavor, and most of it is eaten with cheese and bread on the side. There are several herbs used during cooking, but the food is rarely spicy hot.

The main herbs used are garlic, onions, oregano, lemon juice, cinnamon, gloves, nutmeg, bay leaves, mint or basil. Common sweeteners are sugar and honey. Salt, sugar, and lemon are used as natural preservatives to extend the shelf life of the food.

Sweet is Sweet and salty is salty!

Sugar is used in coffee and in desserts, but rarely used inside the recipe when cooking a dish. There is a distinction of a food being either sweet as a dessert or salty as a main dish. In American cuisine, we often see adding a tablespoon or more of sugar in any recipe and even on potatoes and meat. Adding sugar on a meat is not seen in Mediterranean cuisine. Adding unnecessary and excessive sugars in the diet is implicated in many chronic diseases and metabolic syndromes that lead to diabetes and its complications. Corn syrup, a common unhealthy additive in American food, is never seen in Mediterranean cuisine. Honey is used more often than sugar in Greece. Honey is used inside drinks, desserts and with yogurt.

Example of a weekly Mediterranean menu

Monday:

Breakfast:
Strong coffee, water
cookie

Lunch:
Greek salad with Spanakopita
Lemonade

Afternoon break
1-2 shot glasses ouzo
Poikilia: salami, cheese, olives

Dinner
Tea
1-2 rusks with hard cheese
Greek yogurt with honey and walnuts
Apple, water

Tuesday:

Breakfast:
Coffee and a cookie
juice, water

Lunch:
Gyro and French fries
Orangeade, water

Morning snack: cheese pie
Evening snack: Baklava, Frappe, water

Dinner:
Lentil soup, kouloura & cheese
Tea, water

Wed:

Breakfast:
Fruit and bread with butter
Coffee

Lunch
Stuffed peppers with bread
Beer

Dinner
Chamomile and a rusk with cheese
Yogurt, walnuts and honey, orange
water

Thursday:

Breakfast: coffee and a cookie

Snack:
Spanakopita, grapes, lemonade

Lunch:
Stuffed zucchini, cheese, kouloura
Lemonade

Dinner:
Fava peas, olives, feta, bread
2 glasses of Red wine
Fresh figs, water

Friday

Breakfast: coffee and cookie

Lunch: spanakopita, orangeade

Snack: Kataifi, Frappe, water

Dinner with friends
Moussaka, Greek salad, Greens,
kokoretsi, octopus
4 glasses of retsina wine, water

Saturday

Breakfast:
Coffee, cookie

Evening with friends:
Ouzo, poikilia, smelts

Lunch:
3-4 Souvlaki (meat on the stick)
bread, salad, beer

Dinner with friends:
At tavern with dancing
Roasted chicken with oven
potatoes
dolmadakia, tzatziki, skordalia,
beer
Milk pie

Sunday:

Breakfast
Coffee and pasteli

Dinner
Giant Beans, Feta, taramosalad
(roe fish), bread
Water, tart cherry juice
Mandarin

Lunch:
Grilled Fish, zucchini fritters,
eggplant spread, bread, Wine

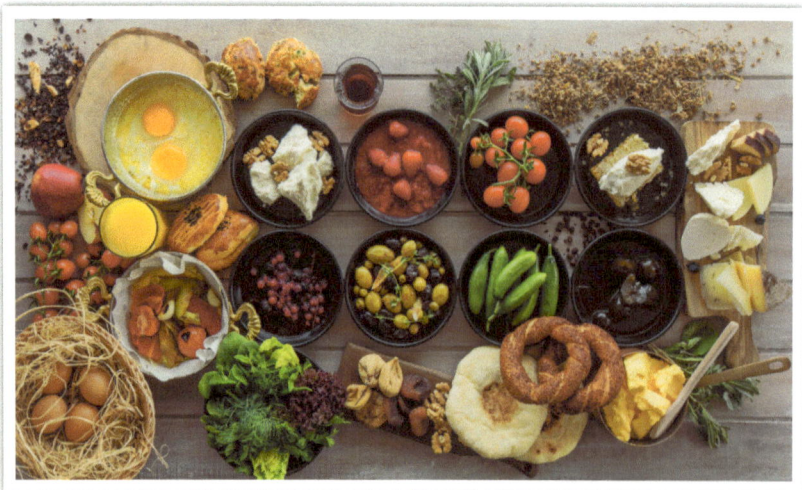

Therapeutic benefits of ingredients found in Med-Diet

The Greek Diet can be seen as "therapeutic," because of its incorporation of herbs in their foods. Cinnamon, garlic, oregano, cloves, olive oil, parsley, basil, mint and lemons are some ingredients rich in nutrients touted for their health benefits. It is not uncommon to see those ingredients at your local health food store, and even prescribed by some "leading-edge" physicians at therapeutic doses for their health benefits. Those supplements have their humble beginnings founded from the Mediterranean cuisine.

Food and herbs have been used as medicine and wellness for thousands of years. Not surprisingly, many herbs and foods have chemicals (vitamins & minerals) that are used by the body to process several chemical reactions that the body needs for repair and to establish homeostasis. Recently there has been an explosion of scientific information based on studies, clinical use and clinical reviews. That explosion has created a new branch of medicine called naturopathic medicine, which deals with integrative medicine based on evidence, science and effectiveness of herbs, supplements, pharmaceutical and natural therapeutics. Traditionally, the majority of medications derived from natural plants, glands, fungus and organisms. Even though many studies have examined extracts and supplements, it brings an understanding to the therapeutic benefits of good nutrition, using herbs and nutrient packed foods.

The following reference section of my publication was taken from various sources such as "Natural Medicines Comprehensive Database. Jellin JM, Gregory PJ, et al. Natural Medicines. Accessed www.NaturalMedicines.com on [11/23/2016] Therapeutic Research Center; 2017" HerbMed Pro, Healthnotes, and pubmed.

The studies are numerous, but I have included only few to validate the value of nutritious foods.

Therapeutic effects of nutrients, and their research
(aka: Science Talk)

Cinnamon (Cassia Cinnamon)

There are three different types of cinnamon, but the most common cinnamon sold in North America is cassia cinnamon

When consumed orally, cinnamon is a carminative and a blood sugar regulating nutrient. Cinnamon as a supplement is used therapeutically for help with diabetes, flatulence, gastrointestinal spasms, nausea and vomiting, diarrhea, infections, the common cold, and loss of appetite. It has also been used for impotence, enuresis, joint pain, menopausal symptoms, amenorrhea, and as an abortifacient. Topically, cinnamon has a use as a mosquito repellent.

Mechanism of Action

Cassia cinnamon contains a wide range of coumarin concentrations that has a blood thinning effect, which can be beneficial against pro-inflammatory actions that leads to blood thickening. In addition, coumarin is an edema modifier by stimulating macrophages to degrade extracellular albumin. There are several terpenoids constituents in cinnamon, such as eugenol and cinnamaldehyde that are believed to account for cinnamon's medicinal effects.

The cinnamon constituent cinnamaldehyde, has antibacterial activity and other related compounds that might have some activity against some human solid tumor cells; by modulating the immune system. Polyphenolic polymers such as hydroxychalcone in cinnamon, can increase insulin sensitivity, which may improve blood glucose control, and lipid levels helping with diabetes. Other polymers isolated from cassia cinnamon also affect other antioxidant activity.

Studies & References:

Int J Immunopharmacol. 1998 Nov;20(11):643-60. Cinnamaldehyde inhibits lymphocyte proliferation and modulates T-cell differentiation. Koh WS1, Yoon SY, Kwon BM, Jeong TC, Nam KS, Han MY.

J Agric Food Chem. 1998 Jan 19;46(1):8-12. Growth-Inhibiting Effects of Cinnamomum cassia Bark-Derived Materials on Human Intestinal Bacteria. Lee HS1, Ahn YJ.

Arch Pharm Res. 1998 Apr;21(2):147-52. Synthesis and in vitro cytotoxicity of cinnamaldehydes to human solid tumor cells. Kwon BM1, Lee SH, Choi SU, Park SH, Lee CO, Cho YK, Sung ND, Bok SH.

J Agric Food Chem. 2004 Jan 14;52(1):65-70. Isolation and characterization of polyphenol type-A polymers from cinnamon with insulin-like biological activity. Anderson RA1, Broadhurst CL, Polansky MM, Schmidt WF, Khan A, Flanagan VP, Schoene NW, Graves DJ.

Horm Res. 1998 Sep;50(3):177-82. Regulation of PTP-1 and insulin receptor kinase by fractions from cinnamon: implications for cinnamon regulation of insulin signalling.

Imparl-Radosevich J1, Deas S, Polansky MM, Baedke DA, Ingebritsen TS, Anderson RA, Graves DJ.

J Agric Food Chem. 2004 Jan 14;52(1):65-70. Isolation and characterization of polyphenol type-A polymers from cinnamon with insulin-like biological activity. Anderson RA1, Broadhurst CL, Polansky MM, Schmidt WF, Khan A, Flanagan VP, Schoene NW, Graves DJ.

CLOVE (Syzygium aromaticum)

Cloves are the unopened pink flower buds of the evergreen clove tree, and have a strong, warm, sweet and aromatic taste and smell. The expert panel German Commission E has approved the use of clove as a topical antiseptic and anesthetic.

Uses:

When taken orally, clove is a carminative and used for dyspepsia, flatulence, nausea, and vomiting, halitosis, tooth pain and as an expectorant. A topical preparation (SS-cream) for treating premature ejaculation, uses clove in combination with other ingredients to get the desired therapeutic effect.

Mechanisms of Action

Eugenol, a volatile oil extracted from clove, is believed, to be responsible for many of the therapeutic effects of clove. Clove and its extract or oil has so many document studies that makes this herb very impressive.

- Analgesic/anesthetic effects: "a randomized trial found that a homemade clove gel is as effective as an oral anesthetic benzocaine 20% gel". The clove component eugenol can inhibit prostaglandin biosynthesis and thereby depress pain sensory receptors.
  (Alqareer, A., Alyahya, A., and Andersson, L. The effect of clove and benzocaine versus placebo as topical anesthetics. J Dent 2006;34(10):747-750)
- Anthelmintic and anti-parasitic effects: Clove can inhibit parasite growth according to several studies.
- Antibacterial effects: Flower extract of clove ethanol extract has been shown to inhibit the growth of several bacteria, including Helicobacter pylori (Gastric Ulcers bacterium). Oil of clove or eugenol has shown a germicidal effect against many bacteria including Klebsiella pneumoniae, Pseudomonas

aerugenosa, Clostridium perfringes, Escherichia coli, Proteus vulgaris, Saccharomyces cerevisiae, Porphyromonas gingivalis, methicillin-resistant Staphylococcus aureus (MRSA) anti-mycotic-resistant Candida species and five strains of Staphylococcus aureus by decreasing the production of enterotoxin A, enterotoxin B. Eugenol may suppress verocytotoxin of Escherichia coli 0157:H7 which may reduce its virulence.

(Essential Oils and Eugenols Inhibit Biofilm Formation and the Virulence of Escherichia coli O157:H7. Kim YG, Lee JH, Gwon G, Kim SI, Park JG, Lee J. Sci Rep. 2016 Nov 3;6:36377. doi: 10.1038/srep36377).

Anticancer effects: Eugenol or clove oil induces apoptosis (cell death) of cancer cells, including DNA fragmentation and formation of DNA ladders.

- Antidiabetic effects: In animal research, treatment with eugenol for two weeks, following six weeks of untreated diabetes, corrected diabetes-induced vascular and neural complications, a potential therapy for diabetic neuropathy and vasculopathy. *(Nangle, M. R., Gibson, T. M., Cotter, M. A., and Cameron, N. E. Effects of eugenol on nerve and vascular dysfunction in streptozotocin-diabetic rats. Planta Med 2006;72(6):494-500).*
- Antifungal effects: Clove oil is a potent anti-fungal, and exhibits activity against Aspergillus species and other fungal pathogens, including Cryptococcus neoformans, Candida albicans and may have a high inhibitory effect on dermatophytic fungi amongst others. The fungicidal activity was similar with nystatin used as a referenced treatment. *(J Biosci Bioeng. 2016 Nov 18. pii: S1389-1723(16)30309-7. doi: 10.1016/j.jbiosc.2016.09.011).*

In addition, clove and its ingredients have antihistamine properties and anti-inflammatory effects by suppressing cyclooxygenase-2 expression. Other beneficial effects of clove ingredients includes anti-mutagenic (cancer prevention), Antioxidant, anti-parasitic, Antipyretic (reducing fever), antispasmodic, antithrombotic effects by inhibiting platelet aggregation (blood thinning effect) and increasing INR, antiviral, cardiovascular and anti-lipidemic effects. The Hormonal effects are by displacing [(3) H] 17beta-estradiol from isolated alpha- and beta-human estrogen receptors by exerting anti-estrogenic or modulating effects. Eugenol is helping with anxiety by interacting with the GABA receptors.

Some other notable effects:

Sexual enhancement effects: Clove extract oral administration to rats, significantly increased sexual effects and behaviors. In Premature ejaculation, a controlled clinical trial used a multi-ingredient cream preparation containing clove flower, plus Panax ginseng root, Angelica root, Cistanches deserticola, Zanthoxyl species, Torlidis seed, Asiasari root, cinnamon bark, and toad venom (SS Cream), this cream was applied to the glans penis one hour prior to sexual intercourse, the cream was then washed off immediately prior to intercourse. Men suffering from premature ejaculation who were treated with this cream, had a significant improvement in their ejaculatory latency period, compared to those receiving a placebo. Eugenol has a vaso-relaxant effect. *https://www.ncbi.nlm.nih.gov/pubmed/10688090*

Another study, suggested the beneficial effects of herbal toothpaste on gingival bleeding, oral hygiene and microbial variables.

Toothache: (traditional use in Greece) Clove oil and its constituent eugenol have long been used topically for toothache. However, the FDA reclassified eugenol to category III, meaning there is insufficient data to support efficacy. It is best not to use undiluted clove oil directly on membranes but add it on carrier oil.

Studies & References:

Phytother Res. 2007 Dec;21(12):1153-8. Anti-herpes simplex virus activities of Eugenia caryophyllus (Spreng.) Bullock & S. G. Harrison and essential oil, eugenol. Tragoolpua Y1, Jatisatienr A

J Dent. 2006 Nov;34(10):747-50. Epub 2006 Mar 13. The effect of clove and benzocaine versus placebo as topical anesthetics. Alqareer A1, Alyahya A, Andersson L.

Fitoterapia. 2001 Aug;72(6):669-70. Anthelmintic activity of essential oil of Ocimum sanctum and eugenol. Asha MK1, Prashanth D, Murali B, Padmaja R, Amit A.

Biol Pharm Bull. 1998 Sep;21(9):990-2. Anti-Helicobacter pylori activity of herbal medicines.
Bae EA1, Han MJ, Kim NJ, Kim DH.

Cancer Lett. 2005 Jul 8;225(1):41-52. Epub 2004 Dec 15. Eugenol isolated from the essential oil of Eugenia caryophyllata induces a reactive oxygen species-mediated apoptosis in HL-60 human promyelocytic leukemia cells. Yoo CB1, Han KT, Cho KS, Ha J, Park HJ, Nam JH, Kil UH, Lee KT.

Planta Med. 2006 May;72(6):494-500. Effects of eugenol on nerve and vascular dysfunction in streptozotocin-diabetic rats. Nangle MR1, Gibson TM, Cotter MA, Cameron NE.

J Food Prot. 1998 May;61(5):616-9. Control of Aspergillus flavus in maize with plant essential oils and their components. Montes-Belmont R1, Carvajal M.

Pharmacol Res. 1997 Dec;36(6):475-80. Antianaphylactic properties of eugenol. Kim HM1, Lee EH, Kim CY, Chung JG, Kim SH, Lim JP, Shin TY.

Prostaglandins Leukot Essent Fatty Acids. 2006 Jan;74(1):23-7. Epub 2005 Oct 7. Eugenol--the active principle from cloves inhibits 5-lipoxygenase activity and leukotriene-C4 in human PMNL cells. Raghavenra H1, Diwakr BT, Lokesh BR, Naidu KA.

Food Chem Toxicol. 2011 Jul;49(7):1521-9. doi: 10.1016/j.fct.2011.03.043. Epub 2011 Apr 5. Water extracts of cinnamon and clove exhibits potent inhibition of protein glycation and anti-atherosclerotic activity in vitro and in vivo hypolipidemic activity in zebrafish. Jin S1, Cho KH.

J Agric Food Chem. 2001 Aug;49(8):4019-25.
Suppression of chemical mutagen-induced SOS response by alkylphenols from clove (Syzygium aromaticum) in the Salmonella typhimurium TA1535/pSK1002 umu test. Miyazawa M1, Hisama M.

Exp Parasitol. 2007 Jul;116(3):283-90. Epub 2007 Feb 1. Trypanosoma cruzi: activity of essential oils from Achillea millefolium L., Syzygium aromaticum L. and Ocimum basilicum L. on epimastigotes and trypomastigotes. Santoro GF1, Cardoso MG, Guimarães LG, Mendonça LZ, Soares MJ.

Biol Pharm Bull. 2001 Feb;24(2):181-7.
Purification and characterization of antithrombotics from Syzygium aromaticum (L.) MErr. & PERRY.

Lee JI1, Lee HS, Jun WJ, Yu KW, Shin DH, Hong BS, Cho HY, Yang HC.
Ceylon Med J. 2011 Mar;56(1):5-9. A randomized double-blind placebo-controlled study on the effects of herbal toothpaste on gingival bleeding, oral hygiene and microbial variables. Jayashankar S1, Panagoda GJ, Amaratunga EA, Perera K, Rajapakse PS.

Garlic (Allium sativum)

Garlic has been called a "panacea" and it is the most well studied herb. Orally, garlic has been used for possible benefits in cardiovascular disease such as in hypertension, hypotension, hyperlipidemia (including familial), coronary heart disease, atherosclerosis, peripheral arterial disease (PAD), and myocardial infarction. Garlic also has beneficial effects for earaches, chronic fatigue syndrome (CFS), and menstrual disorders. Garlic is also used orally for Helicobacter pylori infection, and gastritis. Garlic is used to prevent several cancers and to treat and prevent prostate cancer and bladder cancer. Other uses include treatment of benign prostatic hyperplasia (BPH), cystic fibrosis, osteoarthritis, allergic rhinitis, traveler's diarrhea, pre-eclampsia, vaginal candidiasis, swine flu, and flu, for prevention of the common cold, and for prevention and treatment of bacterial and fungal infections. Garlic is also used in exercise-induced muscle soreness, fibrocystic breast disease, scleroderma, lead toxicity as a chelator, diarrhea, amoebic and bacterial dysentery, tuberculosis, bloody urine, diphtheria, whooping cough, scalp ringworm, hypersensitive teeth, and vaginal trichomoniasis. Other uses include treatment of any kind of infections.

Mechanism of Action:

Many of the pharmacological effects of garlic are credited to the allicin, ajoene, and alliin, also known as S-allyl-L-cysteine sulfoxide. When the garlic bulb is crushed (traditional way of preparing), ground, or cut, the alliin constituent is converted to allicin (also known as diallylthiosulfinate) by the enzyme alliinas. The process to produce odorless aged garlic extract reduces the alliin content to only 3% of what is typically contained in fresh garlic, and possibly lowers the effectiveness. Why not eat skordalia?

Few studies on garlic:

J Nutr Sci Vitaminol (Tokyo). 1999 Dec;45(6):785-90. Antibacterial activity of garlic powder against Escherichia coli O-157. Sasaki J1, Kita T, Ishita K, Uchisawa H, Matsue H.

Atherosclerosis. 1988 Dec;74(3):247-9.
Effect of dried garlic on blood coagulation, fibrinolysis, platelet aggregation and serum cholesterol levels in patients with hyperlipoproteinemia. Harenberg J1, Giese C, Zimmermann R.

Appl Environ Microbiol. 2001 Jan;67(1):475-80.

Antimicrobial properties of garlic oil against human enteric bacteria: evaluation of methodologies and comparisons with garlic oil sulfides and garlic powder. Ross ZM1, O'Gara EA, Hill DJ, Sleightholme HV, Maslin DJ.

J Int Soc Sports Nutr. 2013 Apr 19;10(1):22. doi: 10.1186/1550-2783-10-22. Eight weeks of supplementation with a multi-ingredient weight loss product Prograde Metabolism™ METABO, enhances body composition, reduces hip and waist girth, and increases energy levels in overweight men and women. Lopez HL1, Ziegenfuss TN, Hofheins JE, Habowski SM, Arent SM, Weir JP, Ferrando AA.

Planta Med. 1992 Oct;58(5):417-23. In vitro virucidal effects of Allium sativum (garlic) extract and compounds. Weber ND1, Andersen DO, North JA, Murray BK, Lawson LD, Hughes BG.

Atherosclerosis. 1999 May;144(1):237-49. The antiatherosclerotic effect of Allium sativum. Koscielny J1, Klüssendorf D, Latza R, Schmitt R, Radtke H, Siegel G, Kiesewetter H.

J Pharm Pharmacol. 1997 Sep;49(9):908-11.
Garlic compounds protect vascular endothelial cells from oxidized low density lipoprotein-induced injury. Ide N1, Lau BH.

J Cardiovasc Pharmacol. 1998 Jun;31(6):904-8.
Changes in platelet function and susceptibility of lipoproteins to oxidation associated with administration of aged garlic extract. Steiner M1, Lin RS.

Planta Med. 2009 Feb;75(3):205-10. doi: 10.1055/s-0028-1088396. Epub 2009 Jan 9. Effect of supplementation with garlic oil on activity of Th1 and Th2 lymphocytes from rats. Liu CT1, Su HM, Lii CK, Sheen LY.

Oregano (Origanum vulgare)

"You are not Greek or Italian unless you eat garlic and oregano"

Orally, oregano can be used for infections of the respiratory tract including flu, the common cold, croup, urinary tract infections and helps with cough, asthma, allergies, sinusitis, and bronchitis. Oregano can be beneficial for gastrointestinal disorders, such as dyspepsia and bloating. Other beneficial effects are seen against intestinal parasites, dysmenorrhea, rheumatoid arthritis, headaches, diabetes, bleeding following tooth extraction, heart conditions, and hyperlipidemia. I have personally used it for a severe headache following a festival hangover by chewing on the flower buds and has beneficially worked within an hour.

Oregano oil has some topical uses that help with acne, dandruff, canker sores, toothache, gum disease, ringworm, athlete's foot, rosacea, muscle and joint pain, varicose veins, insect and spider bites, wounds, and warts.

Mechanism of Action

Oregano contains phenolic monoterpenes, and more than 60 different compounds, with the primary ones being carvacrol and thymol. The applicable parts of oregano used medicinally are the leaves and other aboveground parts. Thymol and carvacrol has antibacterial effects (against Staph. aureus and other microorganisms), tinea and hook worm infections, and has anesthetic and antiseptic properties.

Oregano has anti-bacterial, antifungal, antiviral, and anti-diabetic effects.

Studies & References on Oregano

Hammer KA, Carson CF, Riley TV. Antimicrobial activity of essential oils and other plant extracts. J Appl Microbiol 1999;86:985-90

Kivanc M, Akgul A, Dogan A. Inhibitory and stimulatory effects of cumin, oregano and their essential oils on growth and acid production of Lactobacillus plantarum and Leuconostoc mesenteroides. Int J Food Microbiol 1991;13:81-5.

Akgul A, Kivanc M. Inhibitory effects of selected Turkish spices and oregano components on some foodborne fungi. Int J Food Microbiol 1988;6:263-8.

Benito M, Jorro G, Morales C, et al. Labiatae allergy: systemic reactions due to ingestion of oregano and thyme. Ann Allergy Asthma Immunol 1996;76:416-8.

Ultee A, Gorris LG, Smid EJ. Bactericidal activity of carvacrol towards the food-borne pathogen Bacillus cereus. J Appl Microbiol 1998;85:211-8

Chevallier A. Encyclopedia of Herbal Medicine. 2nd ed. New York, NY: DK Publ, Inc., 2000.

Vimalanathan S, Hudson J. Anti-influenza virus activities of commercial oregano oils and their carriers. J App Pharma Sci 2012;2:214.

Sweet Basil (Ocimum basilicum)

"I call Basil the herb that thinks it's a flower." I often use a supplement of Holy Basil (Ocimum tenuiflorum) in my practice as an anxiolytic, anti-diabetic and to reduce cortisol levels. (Dr. Theo Christodoulakis)

Orally, basil is used for stomach spasms, kidney conditions, to promote blood circulation before and after childbirth, to treat snakebites and insect bites, as an appetite stimulant, anti-flatulent, diuretic, lactation stimulant, gargle-aid and as mouth astringent.

Mechanisms of Action

Constituents may differ depending on the height and the species of the plant. Basil is rich in Eugenol, linalool, monoterpenes, sesquiterpenes and phenylpropane derivatives.

Basil has anti-bacterial activity, anti-cancer effects (Basil-induced increase in glutathione-S-transferase activity may offer anticancer benefits), anti-fungal effects, anti-parasitic, anti-viral, antihypertensive, and antidiabetic effects, among other actions. Sweet basil (Ocimum basilicum) has been studied in humans for acne vulgaris.

Studies & References:

Asia Pac J Clin Nutr. 2008;17(4):558-65. Dietary sources of aldose reductase inhibitors: prospects for alleviating diabetic complications. Saraswat M1, Muthenna P, Suryanarayana P, Petrash JM, Reddy GB.

J Agric Food Chem. 2000 Mar;48(3):849-52. Insulin-like biological activity of culinary and medicinal plant aqueous extracts in vitro. Broadhurst CL1, Polansky MM, Anderson RA.

Hypertens Res. 2010 Jul;33(7):727-30. doi: 10.1038/hr.2010.64. Epub 2010 May 7. Antihypertensive effects of Ocimum basilicum L. (OBL) on blood pressure in renovascular hypertensive rats. Umar A1, Imam G, Yimin W, Kerim P, Tohti I, Berké B, Moore N.

Toxicol Appl Pharmacol. 2010 Jun 1;245(2):179-90. doi: 10.1016/j.taap.2010.02.017. Epub 2010 Mar 11.
Identification of nevadensin as an important herb-based constituent inhibiting estragole bioactivation and physiology-based biokinetic modeling of its possible in vivo effect. Alhusainy W1, Paini A, Punt A, Louisse J, Spenkelink A, Vervoort J, Delatour T, Scholz G, Schilter B, Adams T, van Bladeren PJ, Rietjens.

Nepal Med Coll J. 2008 Sep;10(3):176-9.
Controlled programmed trial of Ocimum sanctum leaf on generalized anxiety disorders.

Bhattacharyya D1, Sur TK, Jana U, Debnath PK.
Pharmacol Res. 1998 Aug;38(2):107-10. Ocimum sanctum leaf extract in the regulation of thyroid function in the male mouse. Panda S1, Kar A.

MINT

(Mentha longifolia, Japanese mint, wild mint, garden mint)

There are 13 to 18 species of mint, and the exact distinction between species is unclear.

Mint is a carminative and orally used for diarrhea and painful menstruation, flatulence, improving gastrointestinal and gallbladder function and gallstones, irritable bowel syndrome (IBS), improving appetite and digestion. Helps with nausea, headaches, has effects as an antiseptic, a local anesthetic, and antispasmodic uses. Use of Japanese mint is contra-indicated in individuals with bile duct obstruction or gallbladder inflammation, possibly due to the concern of creating spasms and worsening the situation.

The major chemical constituents are menthol (40.7%), carvone and menthone (23.4%) and it also includes 1,8-cineole, limonene, beta-pinene and beta-caryophyllene.

Studies & References:

Blumenthal M, ed. The Complete German Commission E Monographs: Therapeutic Guide to Herbal Medicines. Trans. S. Klein. Boston, MA: American Botanical Council, 1998

Leung AY, Foster S. Encyclopedia of Common Natural Ingredients Used in Food, Drugs and Cosmetics. 2nd ed. New York, NY: John Wiley & Sons, 1996.

Phytother Res. 2006 Aug;20(8):619-33. A review of the bioactivity and potential health benefits of peppermint tea (Mentha piperita L.). McKay DL1, Blumberg JB.

BMC Complement Altern Med. 2013 Nov 28;13:338. doi: 10.1186/1472-6882-13-338.

Comparison of the antibacterial activity of essential oils and extracts of medicinal and culinary herbs to investigate potential new treatments for irritable bowel syndrome. Thompson A1, Meah D, Ahmed N, Conniff-Jenkins R, Chileshe E, Phillips CO, Claypole TC, Forman DW, Row PE.

Parsley (Petroselinum crispum)

The most common forms of parsley used for medicinal purposes is Petroselinum crispum (curled leaf parsley) and Petroselinum neapolitanum (Italian parsley, also known as flat-leaf parsley)

When used orally, parsley is beneficial against urinary tract infections (UTIs), kidney stones (nephrolithiasis), gastrointestinal (GI) disorders, such as constipation, jaundice, flatulence, indigestion and colic. Parsley can also help for conditions such as diabetes, cough, asthma, edema, osteoarthritis, anemia, hypertension, prostate conditions, to promote menstrual flow, induce abortion, as an aphrodisiac, and as a breath freshener. Parsley has analgesic, antibacterial, anti-cancer, anti-diabetic, anti-thrombotic, anti-hypertensive, anti-halitosis, anti-osteoporotic, anti-diuretic, iron chelating, laxative and anti-oxidant effects.

There are reports that when used topically, parsley can help for chapped skin, bruises, insect bites, and to stimulate hair growth.

Mechanism of Action

Petroselinum crispum has a relatively high concentration of nutritionally important carotenoid phytonutrients, such as lutein-zeaxanthin and beta-carotene among many other constituents such as flavonols, glycosides, apiol, limonene, furocoumarin, etc. Parsley has analgesic, antibacterial, anticancer, anti-fungal, anti-diabetic, anti-coagulant and antiplatelet, anti-hypertensive, anti-oxidant, anti-osteoporotic and anti-spasmodic effects. It also has diuretic and gastrointestinal effects. According to the American Nutritional Medical Association, the potassium, calcium, phosphorous, and iodine in parsley seed, root and leaf promote the healing of kidney and urinary tract infections.

Studies & References:

J Pharm Biomed Anal. 2006 Jun 7;41(3):683-93. Epub 2006 Mar 7.
Bioactive polyacetylenes in food plants of the Apiaceae family: occurrence, bioactivity and analysis.
Christensen LP1, Brandt K.

Phytother Res. 2007 Feb;21(2):99-112.
Natural products as alternative treatments for metabolic bone disorders and for maintenance of bone health. Putnam SE1, Scutt AM, Bicknell K, Priestley CM, Williamson EM.

J Ethnopharmacol. 2002 Mar;79(3):353-7. Diuretic effect and mechanism of action of parsley.
Kreydiyyeh SI1, Usta J.

Ozcelik F, Yarat A Yanardag R Tunali T. Limited Effects of Parsley (Petroselinum crispum) on Protein Glycation and Glutathione in Lenses of Streptozotocin-Induced Diabetic Rats. Pharmaceutical Biology 2001;39(3):230-234

Bursac, M, Popovic, M, Mitic, R, Kaurinovic, B, and Jakovljevic, V. Effects of parsley (Petroselinum crispum) and celery (Apium graveolens) extracts on induction and sleeping time in mice. 2005;43:780-783.

Int J Mol Sci. 2008 Jun;9(7):1196-206. doi: 10.3390/ijms9071196. Epub 2008 Jul 12.
Tea polyphenols and their roles in cancer prevention and chemotherapy.
Chen D1, Dou QP.

World J Urol. 2002 Nov;20(5):285-93. Epub 2002 Oct 17. Botanical medicines for the urinary tract.

Yarnell E.
Am J Chin Med. 2003;31(5):699-711.
Prevention of experimentally-induced gastric ulcers in rats by an ethanolic extract of "Parsley" Petroselinum crispum. Al-Howiriny T1, Al-Sohaibani M, El-Tahir K, Rafatullah S.

Bay Leaf (Laurus nobilis)

Bay leaves were used in ancient Greece as a symbol of praise and scholarship for distinguished people. When used orally, bay leaf acts as a general stimulant, anti-flatulence and a diaphoretic.

Mechanism of Action

The main active constituents of Laurus nobilis is 1,8-cineole. The oil of Laurus nobilis also consists of: 1,8-cineole, linalool, alpha-terpinyl acetate, methyl eugenol, sabinene, trans-sabinene hydrate, eugenol, alpha-pinene, beta-ocimene, beta-pinene, o-cymene, and p-cymene. Cinnamtannin B-1, a proanthocyanidin, among others.

It has anti-bacterial, anti-cancer, anti-convulsive, anti-diabetic, anti-fungal, anti-viral, ACE inhibitory effects.

Studies & References:

J Med Chem. 2007 Aug 9;50(16):3937-44. Epub 2007 Jun 29.
Characterization of the intracellular mechanisms involved in the antiaggregant properties of cinnamtannin B-1 from bay wood in human platelets. Ben Amor N1, Bouaziz A, Romera-Castillo C, Salido S, Linares-Palomino PJ, Bartegi A, Salido GM, Rosado JA.

Esteban, R., Jimenez, E. T., Jimenez, M. S., Morales, D., Hormaetxe, K., Becerril, J. M., and Garcia-Plazaola, J. I. Dynamics of violaxanthin and lutein epoxide xanthophyll cycles in Lauraceae tree species under field conditions. Tree Physiol 2007;27(10):1407-1414.

Kaileh, M., Berghe, W. V., Boone, E., Essawi, T., and Haegeman, G. Screening of indigenous Palestinian medicinal plants for potential anti-inflammatory and cytotoxic activity. J Ethnopharmacol. 9-25-2007;113(3):510-516.

Loizzo, M. R., Tundis, R., Menichini, F., Saab, A. M., Statti, G. A., and Menichini, F. Cytotoxic activity of essential oils from labiatae and lauraceae families against in vitro human tumor models. Anticancer Res 2007;27(5A):3293-3299

Mycopathologia. 2006 Feb;161(2):119-28. Antimicrobial activities of the essential oils of various plants against tomato late blight disease agent Phytophthora infestans. Soylu EM1, Soylu S, Kurt S.

J Clin Biochem Nutr. 2009 Jan;44(1):52-6. doi: 10.3164/jcbn.08-188. Epub 2008 Dec 27. Bay leaves improve glucose and lipid profile of people with type 2 diabetes. Khan A1, Zaman G, Anderson RA.

Phytomedicine. 2002 Apr;9(3):212-6.
Anticonvulsant activity of the leaf essential oil of Laurus nobilis against pentylenetetrazole- and maximal electroshock-induced seizures. Sayyah M1, Valizadeh J, Kamalinejad M.

Pak J Pharm Sci. 2006 Jul;19(3):214-8.
Bactericidal activity of black pepper, bay leaf, aniseed and coriander against oral isolates. Chaudhry NM1, Tariq P.

J Ethnopharmacol. 2006 Nov 3;108(1):31-7. Epub 2006 Apr 28.
The in vitro screening for acetylcholinesterase inhibition and antioxidant activity of medicinal plants from Portugal. Ferreira A1, Proença C, Serralheiro ML, Araújo ME

Sage (Salvia officinalis)

Every traditional house in Greek culture has some loose leaves of Sage in their kitchen cabinet. Sage tea is used as a tea when a person has symptoms of a cold or flu. There are as many as 900 different species of sage, with Salvia officinalis and Salvia lavandulifolia (Salvia lavandulaefolia) mostly used. Salvia officinalis is more commonly used medicinally.

When used orally, sage is used to increase appetite, for excessive perspiration, difficulty with menses, menopausal symptoms, hot flashes, galactorrhea, reduction of saliva secretion and digestive problems such as flatulence, bloating, diarrhea, gastritis and dyspepsia. It can also help against depression, memory enhancement, Alzheimer's disease and cerebral ischemia.

Mechanism of Action

Sage contains beta-carotene and alpha-tocopherol and selenium. Alpha-thujone makes up 30-65% of the monoterpenes of Salvia officinalis with other constituents such as camphor, 1,8-cineole, alpha- and beta-pinene, and bornyl acetate. Other minor constituents (1% or less), includes limonene, camphene, linalool, terpineol, and others. Sage has anti-bacterial, anti-fungal, anti-diabetic, anti-inflammatory, anti-viral, anti-parasitic, cardiovascular, endocrine (against menopausal symptoms and thyroid) effects. Sage's anti-cancer effects, based on carnosol, a constituent of sage. A study indicated the efficacy of S. officinalis extract in the management of mild to moderate Alzheimer's disease, and another study showed promising positive effects on cognitive function by inhaling the aroma of Sage. Sage has also been shown to inhibit the growth of Helicobacter pylori and Campylobacter jejuni.

Few studies on Sage

*Adv Ther. 2011 Jun;28(6):490-500. doi: 10.1007/s12325-011-0027-z. Epub 2011 May 16.
First time proof of sage's tolerability and efficacy in menopausal women with hot flushes.
Bommer S1, Klein P, Suter A.*

*J Clin Pharm Ther. 2003 Feb;28(1):53-9.
Salvia officinalis extract in the treatment of patients with mild to moderate Alzheimer's
disease: a double blind, randomized and placebo-controlled trial. Akhondzadeh S1,
Noroozian M, Mohammadi M, Ohadinia S, Jamshidi AH, Khani M.*

*Hum Psychopharmacol. 2010 Jul;25(5):388-96. doi: 10.1002/hup.1129.
Differential effects of the aromas of Salvia species on memory and mood.
Moss L1, Rouse M, Wesnes KA, Moss M.*

*Phytother Res. 2010 May;24(5):649-56. doi: 10.1002/ptr.2933.
Investigations into the antibacterial activities of phytotherapeutics against
Helicobacter pylori and Campylobacter jejuni. Cwikla C1, Schmidt K, Matthias A, Bone
KM, Lehmann R, Tiralongo E*

*Nutr Cancer. 2009;61(4):564-71. doi: 10.1080/01635580802710733.
Salvia fruticosa, Salvia officinalis, and rosmarinic acid induce apoptosis and inhibit
proliferation of human colorectal cell lines: the role in MAPK/ERK pathway. Xavier CP1,
Lima CF, Fernandes-Ferreira M, Pereira-Wilson C.*

*Int J Food Microbiol. 2008 Jul 31;125(3):242-51. doi: 10.1016/j.ijfoodmicro.2008.04.005.
Epub 2008 Apr 20. Tunisian Salvia officinalis L. and Schinus molle L. essential oils: their
chemical compositions and their preservative effects against Salmonella inoculated
in minced beef meat.
Hayouni el A1, Chraief I, Abedrabba M, Bouix M, Leveau JY, Mohammed H, Hamdi M*

*Planta Med. 2006 Dec;72(15):1378-82. Epub 2006 Nov 7.
Antiviral effect of aqueous extracts from species of the Lamiaceae family against
Herpes simplex virus type 1 and type 2 in vitro. Nolkemper S1, Reichling J, Stintzing
FC, Carle R, Schnitzler P.*

Roman Chamomile (Chamaemelum nobile)

Traditionally drinking chamomile is used for indigestion, nausea, vomiting, anorexia, and commonly given to colicky babies for a good night sleep. It is also used for morning sickness, painful menstrual periods, flatulence, indigestion associated with mental stress, mucous membrane inflammation, sinusitis, generalized anxiety disorder and rheumatic disorders.

Topically Chamomile is used as an anti-inflammatory and antiseptic as an ointment/cream/gel. Topically is used to treat cracked nipples, sore gums, and for irritations of the skin and mucosa.

Mechanism of Action

Chamomile possesses anti-flatulent, antispasmodic, and sedative properties. Roman chamomile contains the coumarin scopoletin-7-glucoside and several flavonoids, their glycosides (including rutin and volatile oils), and other constituents. Some individuals can be allergic to chamomile due to a sesquiterpene lactone that can trigger an allergy.

Roman chamomile is not identical to German chamomile but both plants are similarly used.

References

Newall CA, Anderson LA, Philpson JD. Herbal Medicine: A Guide for Healthcare Professionals. London, UK: The Pharmaceutical Press, 1996

Gruenwald J, Brendler T, Jaenicke C. PDR for Herbal Medicines. 1st ed. Montvale, NJ: Medical Economics Company, Inc., 1998

Phytomedicine. 2016 Dec 15;23(14):1735-1742. doi: 10.1016/j.phymed.2016.10.012. Epub 2016 Oct 24.

Long-term chamomile (Matricaria chamomilla L.) treatment for generalized anxiety disorder: A randomized clinical trial. Mao JJ1, Xie SX2, Keefe JR3, Soeller I4, Li QS4, Amsterdam JD5.

Phytomedicine. 2016 Dec 15;23(14):1699-1705. doi: 10.1016/j.phymed.2016.10.013. Epub 2016 Oct 24.
Short-term open-label chamomile (Matricaria chamomilla L.) therapy of moderate to severe generalized anxiety disorder.

Keefe JR1, Mao JJ2, Soeller I3, Li QS3, Amsterdam JD4

Olive Oil (Olea europaea)

Olive oil is a "juice" because it derives from the fruit of the olive, and in certain cultures like in Greeks, Italians and Spaniards, it is consumed as such. A person eating a traditional Mediterranean Diet can consume about a half a cup of olive oil a day. Olive oil is the principal source of dietary lipids of the Mediterranean diet. Olive oil is an Omega-9 lipid that acts similar to Omega-3 at the cyclo-oxygenase pathway that decreases arachidonic acid and therefore it decreases inflammation. Many Chronic Diseases are implicated with an increase and chronic inflammation. By adding olive oil in the diet, we are adding anti-inflammatory actions against inflammation in the body. In addition, olive oil is collected from the fruit of the olive and not from the seed. Extraction of the oil from the fruit is done by simple pressure and no heat is required, hence the cold press. Olive oil therefore does not break during the processing and no trans-fats are formed as seen in other "weaker" oils (vegetable, flaxseed oil).

The benefits, uses and mechanics of olive should be a separate book due to its abundance of literature. Orally, olive oil has beneficial effects on cardiovascular disease, hypertension, hypercholesterolemia, and diabetes. Olive oil can also have beneficial effects for breast cancer, rheumatoid arthritis (RA), firming the breasts, treating bile duct and gallbladder inflammation, gallstones, migraines, jaundice and flatulence. It also can be used as a mild laxative. There are some reports that olive oil has been used for firming the sagging breast when applied topically. Olive oil is a rich source of antioxidants and fatty acids that can reverse the damage caused by free radicals and prevent sagging breasts by helping to improve the skin tone and texture. Olive oil has also been used traditionally to moisturize and darken the hair, and moisturize the skin, treating stretch marks due to pregnancy, and for protecting the skin from ultraviolet (UV) damage from the sun. Other uses for olive oil is for softening earwax, ringing ears (tinnitus), pain in the ears, wound dressing when treating minor wounds.

Historically the benefits of olive leaves in the Mediterranean region were known and used for the treatment high blood pressure, inflammation, arthritis and fever. Recently a renew interest in olive leaves is seen world-wide for its uses as an anti-viral in influenza, the common cold, Epstein-Barr Virus (EBV), and other viral conditions. As a supplement, it can work well as a diuretic and antipyretic. The authors of a study described olive leaf as a "reverse transcriptase inhibitor" that help decrease viral load.

The best use for olive oil is in cooking, as a salad oil or even as a dipping sauce.

Mechanism of Action

The composition of olive oil varies with the region. Olive oil has Oleic Acid (85%), a monounsaturated omega-9 fatty acid, Linoleic Acid, a polyunsaturated omega-6 fatty acid and Palmitic Acid a saturated fatty acid. It also has traces of squalene and sterols such as phytosterol and tocosterols (vitamin E). Squalene may be a chemopreventive substance that protects people from cancer. Olive oil polyphenols can protect against oxidation of blood lipids by raising HDL and reducing LDL. Olive oil is an Omega-9 lipid that acts similar to Omega-3 at the cyclo-oxygenase pathway that decreases arachidonic acid and therefore it decreases inflammation. Another study concluded that a slight reduction in saturated fat intake, along with the use of extra-virgin olive oil, markedly lowers daily antihypertensive dosage requirements, possibly through enhanced nitric oxide levels stimulated by polyphenols.

Studies & References:

J Med Food. 2006 Summer;9(2):187-95.
Modulatory effects of resveratrol, citroflavan-3-ol, and plant-derived extracts on oxidative stress in U937 cells. O'Brien NM1, Carpenter R, O'Callaghan YC, O'Grady MN, Kerry JP

Posit Health News. 1998 Fall;(No 17):12-4. A new triple combination therapy. Konlee M.

Diabetes Care. 2000 Oct;23(10):1472-7.
Dietary unsaturated fatty acids in type 2 diabetes: higher levels of postprandial lipoprotein on a linoleic acid-rich sunflower oil diet compared with an oleic acid-rich olive oil diet.

Madigan C1, Ryan M, Owens D, Collins P, Tomkin GH.
Int J Epidemiol. 2002 Apr;31(2):474-80.
Risk of first non-fatal myocardial infarction negatively associated with olive oil consumption: a case-control study in Spain. Fernández-Jarne E1, Martínez-Losa E, Prado-Santamaría M, Brugarolas-Brufau C, Serrano-Martínez M, Martínez-González MA.
Bitler CM, Matt K, Irving M, et al. Olive extract supplement decreases pain and improves daily activities in adults with osteoarthritis and decreases plasma homocysteine in those with rheumatoid arthritis. Nutri Res 2007;27:470-7

Am J Epidemiol. 1986 Dec;124(6):903-15. The diet and 15-year death rate in the seven countries study. Keys A, Menotti A, Karvonen MJ, Aravanis C, Blackburn H, Buzina R, Djordjevic BS, Dontas AS, Fidanza F, Keys MH, et al.

J Hypertens. 1996 Dec;14(12):1483-90. Plasma lipids, erythrocyte membrane lipids and blood pressure of hypertensive women after ingestion of dietary oleic acid from two different sources.
Ruíz-Gutiérrez V1, Muriana FJ, Guerrero A, Cert AM, Villar J.

Arch Intern Med. 2000 Mar 27;160(6):837-42.
Olive oil and reduced need for antihypertensive medications.
Ferrara LA1, Raimondi AS, d'Episcopo L, Guida L, Dello Russo A, Marotta T.

Lemon (Citrus limonum)

Lemons and oranges is the therapy used for scurvy, the vitamin C deficiency. It can also help with the common cold and flu, swine flu, tinnitus, Meniere's disease, and nephrolithiasis (kidney stones). It has also been used as a digestive aid, an anti-inflammatory, a diuretic, and to improve vascular permeability.

Mechanisms of action:

Bioflavonoids contained in lemons, have antioxidant effects and are thought to be responsible for the beneficial effects of lemons. Other Lemon bioflavonoids include diosmin, eriodictyol, hesperidin, neohesperidoside, naringenin, eriocitrin, neodiosmin, rutinoside, chrysoeriol, isorhamnetin, limocitrin, limocitrol, isolimocitrol, and others limonenes from citrus oil is the most abundant monoterpene in lemon juice. Some of the coumarins in lemon juice appear to reduce free radical generation by inhibiting the production of nitric oxide. An old study from 1964 suggests that a specific lemon bioflavonoid, eriodictyol glycoside, can increase circulation to the inner ear, helping with Meniere's disease, but no other studies have confirmed this.

Citrate from lemon juice can inhibit the formation of calcium-based kidney stones and seems to increase urinary citrate levels.

References

Trans Am Acad Ophthalmol Otolaryngol. 1964 Jan-Feb;68:45-59. ERIODICTYOL GLYCOSIDE IN MENIERE'S DISEASE. WILLIAMS HL Jr.

J Urol. 1996 Sep;156(3):907-9. Dietary manipulation with lemonade to treat hypocitraturic calcium nephrolithiasis. Seltzer MA1, Low RK, McDonald M, Shami GS, Stoller ML.

Anticancer Res. 2000 Sep- Oct;20(5B):3609-14. Effects of citrus flavonoids on the mutagenicity of heterocyclic amines and on cytochrome P450 1A2 activity. Bear WL1, Teel RW.

Pak J Pharm Sci. 2016 May;29(3):843-52. Anti-inflammatory effects of Citrus sinensis L., Citrus paradisi L. and their combinations. Khan RA1, Mallick N1, Feroz Z2.

Urolithiasis. 2016 Feb;44(1):57-63. doi: 10.1007/s00240-015-0843-8. Epub 2015 Dec 8. Treatment of patients with uric acid stones. Heilberg IP1.

Tomato (Solanum lycopersicum)

Tomato, even though there is no conclusive evidence, tomatoes can have potential beneficial effects in reducing the risk of different types of cancer (prostate, breast, cervical, colorectal, gastric), asthma, cardiovascular disease, hypertension, cataracts, osteoarthritis, the common cold, chills, and digestive disorders. Decreased serum or tissue lycopene concentrations are associated with an increased risk of prostate cancer

Tomatoes have a major dietary source of the carotenoid and lycopene. Several studies have studied the effects of different forms of lycopene, but contradictory evidence seem to overshadow the benefits.

Studies & References:

Cancer Res. 1999 Mar 15;59(6):1225-30.
Lower prostate cancer risk in men with elevated plasma lycopene levels: results of a prospective analysis. Gann PH1, Ma J, Giovannucci E, Willett W, Sacks FM, Hennekens CH, Stampfer MJ.

Cancer Epidemiol Biomarkers Prev. 1996 Oct;5(10):823-33.
cis-trans lycopene isomers, carotenoids, and retinol in the human prostate.
Clinton SK1, Emenhiser C, Schwartz SJ, Bostwick DG, Williams AW, Moore BJ, Erdman JW Jr.

J Nutr. 2003 Jul;133(7):2336-41.Dietary lycopene, tomato-based food products and cardiovascular disease in women. Sesso HD1, Liu S, Gaziano JM, Buring JE.

Ann Epidemiol. 1996 Jan;6(1):41-6. Food and nutrient intake and risk of cataract. Tavani A1, Negri E, La Vecchia C.

J Natl Cancer Inst. 1999 Feb 17;91(4):317-31. Tomatoes, tomato-based products, lycopene, and cancer: review of the epidemiologic literature. Giovannucci E1.

Onion Allium cepa

Orally, onion is used for loss of appetite, for treating dyspepsia, fever, colds, cough, bronchitis, hypertension, preventing atherosclerosis, angina, diabetes, allergies, and asthma. It has antibacterial effects on Gram-negative and Gram-positive bacteria including Staph. aureus, Pseudomonas aeruginosa, Salmonella spp., and Shigella dysenteriae. Epidemiological studies indicate that onions or onion extracts prevents cancer including gastrointestinal cancer, ovarian cancer, and skin cancer. In another animal study it exerted antidepressant effects.

Onion contains flavonoids such as myricetin, quercetin, kaempferol, luteolin, apigenin, rutin, isorhamnetin, phenolic acids, allicepin, organic sulfur compounds and steroidal saponins.

Onion is also a source of vitamin B6, calcium, magnesium, phosphorus, lignans and Thiothamine. Allicepin, is an antifungal peptide from onion bulbs

Studies & References:

Nat Prod Rep. 2005 Jun;22(3):351-68. Epub 2005 May 10.
Bioactive S-alk(en)yl cysteine sulfoxide metabolites in the genus Allium: the chemistry of potential therapeutic agents. Rose P1, Whiteman M, Moore PK, Zhu YZ.

Int J Food Sci Nutr. 2005 Sep;56(6):399-414.
Plant foods in the management of diabetes mellitus: spices as beneficial antidiabetic food adjuncts. Srinivasan K1.

Appl Microbiol. 1969 Jun;17(6):903-5.
Death of Salmonella typhimurium and Escherichia coli in the presence of freshly reconstituted dehydrated garlic and onion. Johnson MG, Vaughn RH.

Pharmazie. 1987 Oct;42(10):687-8.Antibacterial activity of species of the genus Allium. Didry N1, Pinkas M, Dubreuil L.

Mutat Res. 2004 Nov 2;555(1-2):121-31. Signal transduction pathways leading to cell cycle arrest and apoptosis induction in cancer cells by Allium vegetable-derived organosulfur compounds: a review. Herman-Antosiewicz A1, Singh SV.

Biosci Biotechnol Biochem. 2008 Jan;72(1):94-100. Epub 2008 Jan 7.
Antidepressant-like effect of onion (Allium cepa L.) powder in a rat behavioral model of depression. Sakakibara H1, Yoshino S, Kawai Y, Terao J.

J Med Food. 2009 Jun;12(3):552-60. doi: 10.1089/jmf.2008.1071.
The antidiabetic effect of onion and garlic in experimental diabetic rats: meta-analysis. Kook S1, Kim GH, Choi K.

J Pept Sci. 2004 Mar;10(3):173-7.
Isolation of allicepin, a novel antifungal peptide from onion (Allium cepa) bulbs. Wang HX1, Ng TB.

Arzneimittelforschung. 2001 Feb;51(2):104-11.
Effects of an onion-olive oil maceration product containing essential ingredients of the Mediterranean diet on blood pressure and blood fluidity.
Mayer B1, Kalus U, Grigorov A, Pindur G, Jung F, Radtke H, Bachmann K, Mrowietz C, Koscielny J, Wenzel E, Kiesewetter H.

English Walnut (Juglans regia)

Orally, English walnut fruit is beneficial for hypertension and lowering cholesterol. The hull of the English walnut is used to treat gastrointestinal mucous membrane inflammation and in TCM (Traditional Chinese Medicine) to treat "blood poisoning" and as a "blood purifier" to remove undesirable agents from the blood. The leaf can be used orally for treating diarrhea, and parasites.

In foods, English walnut is commonly consumed, usually as a snack, in baking and in salads.

Mechanism of Action

The relevant parts of the English walnut are the fruit, hull, and leaf. The walnut fruit (the "nut") comprises high amounts of the polyunsaturated fatty acids, linoleic acid (an omega-6 fatty acid) and alpha-linolenic acid (an omega-3 fatty acid). It also contains other noteworthy amounts of fiber, phosphorus, potassium, folate, vitamin E (gamma-tocopherol), ellagic acid and significant amounts of arginine, a precursor amino acid of the endogenous vasodilator nitric oxide (NO). The walnut hulls and leaves contain juglone and plumbagin, which have astringent, antibacterial, antiviral and antifungal properties. In Greece, the use of the hull and the leaves is not common.

Clinical research advocates English walnut fruit can lower the risk of cardiovascular disease by lowering total and low-density lipoprotein (LDL) cholesterol and might improve endothelial function, which might be beneficial in preventing atherosclerosis.

Studies & References:

J Nutr. 2002 May;132(5):1062S-1101S. The scientific evidence for a beneficial health relationship between walnuts and coronary heart disease. Feldman EB1.

J Nutr. 2001 Nov;131(11):2837-42.
Walnut polyphenolics inhibit in vitro human plasma and LDL oxidation.
Anderson KJ1, Teuber SS, Gobeille A, Cremin P, Waterhouse AL, Steinberg FM.

N Engl J Med. 1993 Mar 4;328(9):603-7.
Effects of walnuts on serum lipid levels and blood pressure in normal men.
Sabaté J1, Fraser GE, Burke K, Knutsen SF, Bennett H, Lindsted KD.

Diabetes Care. 2004 Dec;27(12):2777-83. Including walnuts in a low-fat/modified-fat diet improves HDL cholesterol-to-total cholesterol ratios in patients with type 2 diabetes. Tapsell LC1, Gillen LJ, Patch CS, Batterham M, Owen A, Baré M, Kennedy M.

Almond (Prunus amygdalus)

Orally, sweet almonds can be used as a mild laxative, and as a remedy for cancer of the bladder, breast, mouth, spleen, and uterus.

Mechanism of Action

Almond is a nutritionally dense food which means it includes significant amounts of B vitamins, folate, vitamin E, and the essential minerals calcium, iron, magnesium, manganese, potassium, phosphorus, and zinc. It is rich in dietary fiber, monounsaturated fats, and polyunsaturated fats, fats that potentially may lower LDL cholesterol. In addition, it contains phytosterols such as beta-sitosterol, stigmasterol, campesterol, sitostanol, and campestanol, which have been associated with cholesterol-lowering properties.

Almonds were found to have highly significant hypoglycemic effects, the Almond is the symbol of fertility and studies have found that almond extracts increase sperm count and sperm motility in rats, with no evidence of spermatotoxicity.

Point of interest: Almonds and peanuts are susceptible to aflatoxin-producing molds and should be pasteurized before consumed. Aflatoxins are potent carcinogenic chemicals.

Studies & References:

J Am Coll Nutr. 1998 Jun;17(3):285-90.
Nuts and plasma lipids: an almond-based diet lowers LDL-C while preserving HDL-C.
Spiller GA1, Jenkins DA, Bosello O, Gates JE, Cragen LN, Bruce B.

J Am Coll Nutr. 1992 Apr;11(2):126-30.
Effect of a diet high in monounsaturated fat from almonds on plasma cholesterol and lipoproteins.
Spiller GA1, Jenkins DJ, Cragen LN, Gates JE, Bosello O, Berra K, Rudd C, Stevenson M, Superko R.

Qureshi S, Shah AH, Tariq M, and et al. Studies on herbal aphrodisiacs used in Arab systems of medicine. Amer J Chin Med 1989;17(1-2):57-63

Indian J Physiol Pharmacol. 1997 Oct;41(4):383-9. Effect of Prunus amygdalus seeds on lipid profile.
Teotia S1, Singh M, Pant MC.

Coffee (Coffea arabica, C. robusta)

Orally, coffee increases mental alertness, helps with physical fatigue, mental and physical performance. In high doses, coffee is a laxative and has a diuretic effect. There are several studies that have shown oral coffee consumption to have beneficial effects for prevention or a reduction in the clinical expression of Parkinson's disease, symptomatic gallstone disease, type 2 diabetes, gastrointestinal cancer, lung cancer, breast cancer, headache, hypotension, weight loss, and attention deficit-hyperactivity disorder (ADHD). Some epidemiologic studies show, that drinking coffee has been associated with a decreased risk of gout while others have shown an increased risk of Gout. Many pharmaceutical medications can interact with coffee, so be sure to check with a good physician that knows your medical history.

Mechanism of actions

Coffee contains caffeine, chlorogenic acid, caffeol, diterpenes and polyphenols including the phytoestrogens formononetin and the lignan precursor secoisolariciresinol. The caffeine constituent acts as a central nervous system (CNS) stimulant, that increases heart rate and contractility, increases blood pressure, stimulates gastric acid secretion, causes diuresis, relaxes extracerebral vascular and bronchial smooth muscle, and stimulates the release of catecholamines. Caffeine also prevents platelet aggregation and increases the fibrinolytic activity in blood, which moderately thins the blood that counteracts the inflammatory action of thickening the blood seen in chronic diseases. Coffee has properties that might be beneficial in preventing cardiovascular disease and others that might increase your risk, such as rising LDL and Homocysteine. This effect is probably due to genetic variations of the individuals of a population.

Evidence suggests that long-term consumption of moderate coffee consumption is associated with a lower risk of developing type 2 diabetes, and diabetes in young to middle-aged women. Moderate consumption was classified at about two or more cups of coffee a day. The mechanism is not clear but coffee constituents may beneficially affect insulin sensitivity.

In another study, consumption of a "boiled Greek type of coffee" is associated with improved endothelial function (the Ikaria study). Endothelial dysfunction can result or contribute to several disease processes including but not limited to coronary heart disease. Endothelial dysfunction can be caused by many environmental factors such as pollution, smoking, shift working, and many other unhealthy factors. By improving endothelial factors, we can reduce many chronic diseases. Endothelial dysfunction probably is caused by many factors.

Other researchers found a significant inverse relationship between the incidence of Parkinson's and caffeine use among the Japanese. Non-coffee drinkers were three times as likely to develop Parkinson's as those who did drink coffee.

In another study, coffee consumption is associated with an increase in cardiac wave reflections but not with an increase in aortic stiffness in hypertensive adults, contradicting previous notions of harmful aortic stiffness due to coffee consumption. Excessive doses of caffeine can cause massive catecholamine release and subsequent sinus tachycardia, metabolic acidosis, hyperglycemia, and ketosis. People experiencing heart palpitations with drinking coffee should moderate their coffee consumption.

Studies & References:

Van Dam RM, Hu FB. Coffee consumption and risk of type 2 diabetes: a systematic review. JAMA. July 6, 2005; 294(1):97-104.

Vasc Med. 2013 Apr;18(2):55-62. doi: 10.1177/1358863X13480258. Epub 2013 Mar 18. Consumption of a boiled Greek type of coffee is associated with improved endothelial function: the Ikaria study. Siasos G1, Oikonomou E, Chrysohoou C, Tousoulis D, Panagiotakos D, Zaromitidou M, Zisimos K, Kokkou E, Marinos G, Papavassiliou AG, Pitsavos C, Stefanadis C.

Coffee May Lower Risk of Parkinson's Disease British Medical Journal. Volume 320 3 June 2000,

JAMA. 2000 May 24-31;283(20):2674-9.
Association of coffee and caffeine intake with the risk of Parkinson disease.
Ross GW1, Abbott RD, Petrovitch H, Morens DM, Grandinetti A, Tung KH, Tanner CM, Masaki KH, Blanchette PL, Curb JD, Popper JS, White LR.

Nolan L. The world's favorite beverage - coffee - and health Journal of Herbs, Spices, & Medicinal Plants. 2001;8(2/3):119-15

Arthritis Rheum. 2007 Jun;56(6):2049-55. Coffee consumption and risk of incident gout in men: a prospective study. Choi HK1, Willett W, Curhan G.

Thromb Diath Haemorrh. 1967 Dec 31;18(3-4):670-3. Inhibition and reversal of platelet aggregation by methyl xanthines. Ardlie NG, Glew G, Schultz BG, Schwartz CJ.

Atherosclerosis. 1977 Feb;26(2):255-60. Short-term effect of coffee on blood fibrinolytic activity in healthy adults. Samarrae WA, Truswell AS.

Honey (Apis mellifera)

The therapeutic properties of honey are in promoting rapid wound healing, antibacterial effects, immune stimulation, anti-lipidemic effects, reducing edema and inflammation, clean necrotic tissue and stimulate tissue regeneration. The anti-inflammatory and anti-bacterial properties of honey may be due to inflammatory cytokine release in surrounding tissue cells, such as monocytes and macrophages. The strong antibacterial and anti-fungal effects of honey is suggested to be due to the phenolic compounds and the exerting prebiotic effects via decreasing prostaglandin levels, thus, increasing nitric oxide levels. There are also some clinical reports of the beneficial effects of honey against allergies and asthma.

Local honey has been used for the desensitization of allergies in oral immunotherapy. The theory is that flying bees carry small amount of pollen from different plants, and therefore, found inside the honey. When humans chronically ingest honey, they are ingesting these possible allergens. This action can potentially desensitize individuals for certain environmental allergies. Even though scientific studies might not able to confirm this, at this time, the anecdotal reports are enough to promote the consumption of honey, instead of other synthetic sweeteners.

Honey consists of phenolic constituents such as quercetin, caffeic acid, caffeic acid phenethyl ester (CAPE), chrysin, acacetin, pinocembrin, pinobanksin, apigenin, kaempferol, and galangin

Studies & References

Recent Pat Antiinfect Drug Discov. 2009 Nov;4(3):206-13. Rediscovering the antibiotics of the hive.
Boukraâ L1, Sulaiman SA.

J Periodontol. 2012 Sep;83(9):1116-21. doi: 10.1902/jop.2012.110461. Epub 2012 Feb 6. A comparative evaluation of the antibacterial efficacy of honey in vitro and antiplaque efficacy in a 4-day plaque regrowth model in vivo: preliminary results. Aparna S1, Srirangarajan S, Malgi V, Setlur KP, Shashidhar R, Setty S, Thakur S.

J Med Food. 2011 Oct;14(10):1079-96. doi: 10.1089/jmf.2010.0161. Epub 2011 Aug 22. Honey and microbial infections: a review supporting the use of honey for microbial control.
Al-Waili NS1, Salom K, Butler G, Al Ghamdi AA.

J Med Food. 2011 May;14(5):551-5. doi: 10.1089/jmf.2010.0082. Epub 2010 Dec 27. Effect of honey on 50% complement hemolytic activity in infants with protein energy malnutrition: a randomized controlled pilot study. Abdulrhman MA1, Nassar MF, Mostafa HW, El-Khayat ZA, Abu El Naga MW.

Cytokine. 2001 May 21;14(4):240-2. Stimulation of TNF-alpha release in monocytes by honey.
Tonks A1, Cooper RA, Price AJ, Molan PC, Jones KP.

ScientificWorldJournal. 2008 Apr 20;8:463-9. doi: 10.1100/tsw.2008.64. Natural honey and cardiovascular risk factors; effects on blood glucose, cholesterol, triacylglycerole, CRP, and body weight compared with sucrose. Yaghoobi N1, Al-Waili N, Ghayour-Mobarhan M, Parizadeh SM, Abasalti Z, Yaghoobi Z, Yaghoobi F, Esmaeili H, Kazemi-Bajestani SM, Aghasizadeh R, Saloom KY, Ferns GA.

J Med Food. 2004 Spring;7(1):100-7. Al-Waili NS1. Natural honey lowers plasma glucose, C-reactive protein, homocysteine, and blood lipids in healthy, diabetic, and hyperlipidemic subjects: comparison with dextrose and sucrose.

Mastic (Pistacia lentiscus)

Therapeutically, mastic has an antibacterial action used for dyspepsia, gastric and duodenal ulcers, respiratory conditions, muscle aches, and to improve circulation. It is also used for bacterial and fungal infections. Mastic gum has bactericidal activity on H. pylori in vivo, successful treatment of Crohn's disease and periodontitis. There is a good prescription type of supplement by Allergy Research that I commonly use for patients with H. pylori infections. Mastic also has anti-helmitic, anti-parasitic, anti-fungal, anti-neoplastic, anti-diabetic, and anti-inflammatory effects. In dentistry, mastic resin was used as a material for fillings. The resin of mastic in chewing gums release substances that freshen the breath and tighten the gums.

Even Hippocrates, the father of medicine (350 BC) recommended Mastic, stating that it is good for the prevention of digestive problems and colds.

Mechanism of Action

The main components of Pistacia lenticus were found to be: Alpha-pinene, beta-myrcene, beta-pinene, limonene, beta-caryophyllene, pinene, myrcene, trans-caryophyllene, and germacrene D as well as other trace components such as palmitic, oleic, and linoleic fatty acids.

Studies & References:

J Ethnopharmacol. 2010 Feb 3;127(2):205-9. doi: 10.1016/j.jep.2009.11.021. Epub 2009 Dec 2.
Is Chios mastic gum effective in the treatment of functional dyspepsia? A prospective randomised double-blind placebo controlled trial. Dabos KJ1, Sfika E, Vlatta LJ, Frantzi D, Amygdalos GI, Giannikopoulos G.

Phytomedicine. 2010 Mar;17(3-4):296-9. doi: 10.1016/j.phymed.2009.09.010. Epub 2009 Oct 29.
The effect of mastic gum on Helicobacter pylori: a randomized pilot study. Dabos KJ1, Sfika E, Vlatta LJ, Giannikopoulos G.

World J Gastroenterol. 2007 Feb 7;13(5):748-53.
Chios mastic treatment of patients with active Crohn's disease.
Kaliora AC1, Stathopoulou MG, Triantafillidis JK, Dedoussis GV, Andrikopoulos NK.

J Agric Food Chem. 2005 Oct 5;53(20):7681-5.
Chemical composition and antibacterial activity of the essential oil and the gum of Pistacia lentiscus Var. chia. Koutsoudaki C1, Krsek M, Rodger A.

Nutr Cancer. 2009;61(5):640-8. doi: 10.1080/01635580902825647.
Protective effects of mastic oil from Pistacia lentiscus variation chia against experimental growth of lewis lung carcinoma. Magkouta S1, Stathopoulos GT, Psallidas I, Papapetropoulos A, Kolisis FN, Roussos C, Loutrari H.

Nutr Cancer. 2006;55(1):86-93. Mastic oil from Pistacia lentiscus var. chia inhibits growth and survival of human K562 leukemia cells and attenuates angiogenesis. Loutrari H1, Magkouta S, Pyriochou A, Koika V, Kolisis FN, Papapetropoulos A, Roussos C.

Wine

Wine consists of alcohol and polyphenolic compounds such as trans-resveratrol, proanthocyanidins; anthocyanins; and flavonoids such as quercetin, kaempferol, and catechins.

Moderate alcohol use (one to two drinks per day) reduces the risk of coronary heart disease, atherosclerosis, and myocardial infarction (MI), by approximately 30% to 50% when compared with nondrinkers. Excessive alcohol use increases cardiovascular risks.

One to two alcoholic drinks per day increases high-density lipoprotein (HDL) cholesterol by about 12%, decrease blood pressure, improves cognitive function in the elderly, and may be associated with increased insulin sensitivity and a reduced risk of diabetes

Red wine has higher concentrations of polyphenolic compounds than other alcoholic drinks. The antioxidant properties of these polyphenols may contribute to protection against coronary heart disease by reducing oxidation of LDL cholesterol

References and Studies:

Circulation. 2001 Jan 23;103(3):472-5. AHA Science Advisory: Wine and your heart: a science advisory for healthcare professionals from the Nutrition Committee, Council on Epidemiology and Prevention, and Council on Cardiovascular Nursing of the American Heart Association. Goldberg IJ, Mosca L, Piano MR, Fisher EA; Nutrition Committee, Council on Epidemiology and Prevention, and Council on Cardiovascular Nursing of the American Heart Association.

Clin Chim Acta. 1996 Mar 15;246(1-2):51-7. Alcohol and coronary heart disease: consistent relationship and public health implications. Criqui MH1.

Am J Cardiol. 1997 Aug 15;80(4):416-20.
Red wine, white wine, liquor, beer, and risk for coronary artery disease hospitalization. Klatsky AL1, Armstrong MA, Friedman GD.

Circulation. 1996 Dec 1;94(11):3023-5. Alcohol and heart disease. Pearson TA.

N Engl J Med. 1993 Dec 16;329(25):1829-34. Moderate alcohol intake, increased levels of high-density lipoprotein and its subfractions, and decreased risk of myocardial infarction. Gaziano JM1, Buring JE, Breslow JL, Goldhaber SZ, Rosner B, VanDenburgh M, Willett W, Hennekens CH.

Am J Clin Nutr. 2002 Mar;75(3):593-9. Moderate alcohol consumption lowers risk factors for cardiovascular disease in postmenopausal women fed a controlled diet. Baer DJ1, Judd JT, Clevidence BA, Muesing RA, Campbell WS, Brown ED, Taylor PR.

BMJ. 1995 Mar 4;310(6979):555-9. Prospective study of cigarette smoking, alcohol use, and the risk of diabetes in men. Rimm EB1, Chan J, Stampfer MJ, Colditz GA, Willett WC.

Am J Public Health. 2000 Aug;90(8):1254-9.
A longitudinal study of drinking and cognitive performance in elderly Japanese American men: the Honolulu-Asia Aging Study.
Galanis DJ1, Joseph C, Masaki KH, Petrovitch H, Ross GW, White L.

Br J Psychiatry. 2000 Jul;177:66-71.Long-term predictors of cognitive outcome in a cohort of older people with hypertension. Cervilla JA1, Prince M, Joels S, Lovestone S, Mann A.

Mediterranean Diet, also known as: The Greek Diet

The Mediterranean diet originated in Greece, and specifically, in Crete. Med-Diet is rich in heart-healthy fiber, nutrients and antioxidants that come from grains, legumes, nuts, seafood, vegetables, fruit and unsaturated fats, particularly from olive oil. Wine and coffee also play a beneficial role in this healthy diet.

The Mediterranean diet is being promoted for its beneficial effects against cancer, heart disease, diabetes, weight loss, and overall health.

PREGNANCY: There is insufficient reliable evidence about the safety of the Mediterranean diet in pregnancy. There is no reason to expect safety issues; however, pregnant women should avoid alcohol consumption.

Mechanism of Action

Olive oil, the main fat of the Mediterranean diet, contains a high level of monounsaturated fatty acids, that has antioxidant and anti-inflammatory effects, that protect the body from oxidation by inactivating free radicals. The high portion of monounsaturated fatty acids in olive oil is believed to decrease LDL (bad) cholesterol and increase HDL (good) cholesterol.

The Mediterranean diet includes wine and olive oil which contain tyrosol and caffeic acid. Tyrosol helps to lower cholesterol levels and caffeic acid can have antimitogenic, anticarcinogenic, anti-inflammatory, and immunomodulatory properties.

Population studies show, that a number of cancers, such as cancer of the large bowel and breast, are less frequent in Mediterranean countries than in northern Europe.

Med Diet Studies & References:

Healthy dietary patterns and incidence of biliary tract and gallbladder cancer in a prospective study of women and men. Larsson SC, Håkansson N, Wolk A.
Eur J Cancer. 2016 Nov 18;70:42-47. doi: 10.1016/j.ejca.2016.10.012. [Epub ahead of print]

Good adherence to Mediterranean diet can prevent gastrointestinal symptoms: A survey from Southern Italy.
Zito FP, Polese B, Vozzella L, Gala A, Genovese D, Verlezza V, Medugno F, Santini A, Barrea L, Cargiolli M, Andreozzi P, Sarnelli G, Cuomo R. World J Gastrointest Pharmacol Ther. 2016 Nov 6;7(4):564-571

Higher adherence to the Mediterranean diet is associated with lower levels of D-dimer: findings from the MOLI-SANI study.
Di Castelnuovo A, Bonaccio M, De Curtis A, Costanzo S, Persichillo M, de Gaetano G, Donati MB, Iacoviello L; MOLI-SANI investigators.. Haematologica. 2016 Oct 20. pii: haematol.2016.156331. [Epub ahead of print] No abstract available.

Mediterranean Diet Score and Its Association with Age-Related Macular Degeneration: The European Eye Study.
Hogg RE, Woodside JV, McGrath A, Young IS, Vioque JL, Chakravarthy U, de Jong PT, Rahu M, Seland J, Soubrane G, Tomazzoli L, Topouzis F, Fletcher AE.
Ophthalmology. 2016 Nov 5. pii: S0161-6420(16)31351-3. doi: 10.1016/j. ophtha.2016.09.019. [Epub ahead of print]

Mediterranean diet could cut cardiovascular disease risk. Nurs Stand. 2016 Oct 5;31(6):17.

Adherence to the Mediterranean diet is associated with better quality of life: data from the Osteoarthritis Initiative. Veronese N, Stubbs B, Noale M, Solmi M, Luchini C, Maggi S.
Am J Clin Nutr. 2016 Nov;104(5):1403-1409.

Short-term Exposure to a Mediterranean Environment Influences Attitudes and Dietary Profile in U.S. College Students: The Mediterranean Diet in Americans (A-MED-AME) Pilot Study.
Petroka K, Dinu M, Hoover C, Casini A, Sofi F.. J Am Coll Nutr. 2016 Sep-Oct;35(7):621-626.

Polyphenol-rich virgin olive oil reduces insulin resistance and liver inflammation and improves mitochondrial dysfunction in high fat diet fed rats.
Lama A, Pirozzi C, Mollica MP, Trinchese G, Guida FD, Cavaliere G, Calignano A, Raso GM, Canani RB, Meli R.
Mol Nutr Food Res. 2016 Oct 29. doi: 10.1002/mnfr.201600418

Mediterranean diets supplemented with virgin olive oil and nuts enhance plasmatic antioxidant capabilities and decrease xanthine oxidase activity in people with metabolic syndrome: The PREDIMED study.
Sureda A, Bibiloni MD, Martorell M, Buil-Cosiales P, Marti A, Pons A, Tur JA, Martinez-Gonzalez MÁ; PREDIMED Study Investigators.. Mol Nutr Food Res. 2016 Sep 7. doi: 10.1002/mnfr.201600450

Extra virgin olive oil: a key functional food for prevention of immune-inflammatory diseases.
Aparicio-Soto M, Sánchez-Hidalgo M, Rosillo MÁ, Castejón ML, Alarcón-de-la-Lastra C.
Food Funct. 2016 Nov 9;7(11):4492-4505. Review.

Olive polyphenols: new promising agents to combat aging-associated neurodegeneration.
Casamenti F, Stefani M. Expert Rev Neurother. 2016 Oct 20:1-14

Diet Quality-The Greeks Had It Right!
Anderson JJ, Nieman DC. Nutrients. 2016 Oct 14;8(10). pii: E636.

Mediterranean diet and life expectancy; beyond olive oil, fruits, and vegetables.
Martinez-Gonzalez MA, Martin-Calvo N.
Curr Opin Clin Nutr Metab Care. 2016 Nov;19(6):401-407

The anticancer and antiobesity effects of Mediterranean diet.
Kwan HY, Chao X, Su T, Fu X, Tse AK, Fong WF, Yu ZL.
Crit Rev Food Sci Nutr. 2017 Jan 2;57(1):82-94.

Benefits of the Mediterranean diet beyond the Mediterranean Sea and beyond food patterns.
Martínez-González MA. BMC Med. 2016 Oct 14;14(1):157.

Cardioprotective effects of the polyphenol hydroxytyrosol from olive oil.
Tejada S, Pinya S, Del Mar Bibiloni M, Tur JA, Pons A, Sureda A.
Curr Drug Targets. 2016 Oct 5.

Mediterranean diet in UK shows positive effects in study.
Wise J. BMJ. 2016 Sep 28;354:i5286. doi: 10.1136/bmj.i5286

Mediterranean diet, Dietary Approaches to Stop Hypertension (DASH) style diet, and metabolic health in U.S. adults.
Park YM, Steck SE, Fung TT, Zhang J, Hazlett LJ, Han K, Lee SH, Kwon HS, Merchant AT.
Clin Nutr. 2016 Sep 8. pii: S0261-5614(16)30217-5. doi: 10.1016/j.clnu.2016.08.018

Mediterranean Diet, Cognitive Function, and Dementia: A Systematic Review of the Evidence.
Petersson SD, Philippou E.
Adv Nutr. 2016 Sep 15;7(5):889-904. doi: 10.3945/an.116.012138. Review

A breaking down of the Mediterranean diet in the land where it was discovered. A cross sectional survey among the young generation of adolescents in the heart of Cilento, Southern Italy.
Saulle R, Del Prete G, Stelmach-Mardas M, De Giusti M, La Torre G.
Ann Ig. 2016 Sep-Oct;28(5):349-59. doi: 10.7416/ai.2016.2115.

Are 6-8 year old Italian children moving away from the Mediterranean diet?
Zani C, Ceretti E, Grioni S, Viola GC, Donato F, Feretti D, Festa A, Bonizzoni S, Bonetti A, Monarca S, Villarini M, Levorato S, Carducci A, Verani M, Casini B, De Donno A, Grassi T, Bagordo F, Carraro E, Bonetta S, Bonetta S, Gelatti U; MAPEC-LIFE Study Group.. Ann Ig. 2016 Sep-Oct;28(5):339-48. doi: 10.7416/ai.2016.2114

Diet quality and academic achievement: a prospective study among primary school children.
Haapala EA, Eloranta AM, Venäläinen T, Jalkanen H, Poikkeus AM, Ahonen T, Lindi V, Lakka TA. Eur J Nutr. 2016 Sep 9

Sexual Dysfunction
Rev Med Suisse Romande. 2003 Mar;123(3):183-9. Prevention of cardiovascular and degenerative diseases: II. Hormones and/or Mediterranean diet].
Martin-Du Pan R.

J Diabetes Complications. 2016 Nov - Dec;30(8):1519-1524. doi: 10.1016/j. jdiacomp.2016.08.007. Epub 2016 Aug 12. Effects of Mediterranean diet on sexual function in people with newly diagnosed type 2 diabetes: The MÈDITA trial. Maiorino MI1, Bellastella G2, Caputo M3, Castaldo F4, Improta MR5, Giugliano D6, Esposito K7.
Diabetes Care. 2016 Sep;39(9):e143-4. doi: 10.2337/dc16-0910. Epub 2016 Jun 28.
Primary Prevention of Sexual Dysfunction With Mediterranean Diet in Type 2 Diabetes: The MÈDITA Randomized Trial. Maiorino MI1, Bellastella G2, Chiodini P3, Romano O4, Scappaticcio L2, Giugliano D2, Esposito K4.

Int J Impot Res. 2007 Sep-Oct;19(5):486-91. Epub 2007 Aug 2.
Mediterranean diet improves sexual function in women with the metabolic syndrome. Esposito K1, Ciotola M, Giugliano F, Schisano B, Autorino R, Iuliano S, Vietri MT, Cioffi M, De Sio M, Giugliano D.

Public Health Nutr. 2006 Dec;9(8A):1118-20.
Sexual dysfunction and the Mediterranean diet.
Giugliano D1, Giugliano F, Esposito K.

And many more …

Recipes

So, now that you know the science and the benefits of the Mediterranean Diet, are you ready to enjoy some good healthy food?

There are many factors that influence cooking and eating. If at first, the recipe does not come out right, try it again by following the directions, your intuition and improving the techniques a little more closely. Sometimes, it just takes practice.

Believe it or not, water, spices, ingredients, and the type of cookware you use, along with the emotions that you feel while you cook and eat, accompanied by the people surrounding you, influence the taste and the enjoyment of your food.

There are some things you cannot change, and then there are some things **YOU CAN**!

Mouth Watering & Healthful Recipes
To cook you must be inspired!

If you cook for someone you must love them,
If you eat with someone you are loved!

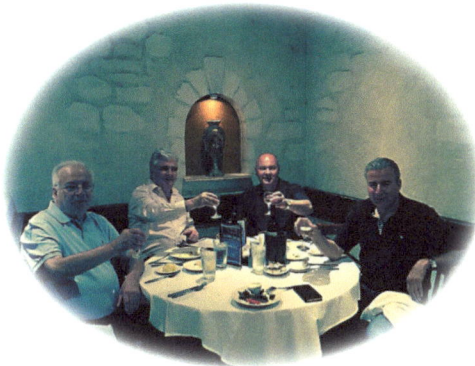

Stuffed zucchini with lemon egg sauce (Avgolemeno)

Healthy, lemony and creamy dish

Ingredients for stuffed zucchini:

4 zucchinis (cut in half and cored) reserve the insides for the stuffing
1 tablespoon olive oil
1 onion (chopped)
4 cloves garlic (chopped)
1-pound ground meat (beef, pork, lamb, etc.)
1/4 cup parsley (chopped)
1/3 cup dill (chopped)
1 tablespoon mint (chopped)
Zest of 1 lemon (zest lemon from the Avgolemono sauce)
1 cup white rice
1 cup chicken stock
2 egg whites (use the ones left over from the Avgolemono sauce)
1 cup chicken stock

See "avgolemono sauce" recipe
Avgolemono is a mixture of egg yolks, lemon juice and broth. It can be used in anything from a sauce to a stew to a soup.

Ingredients for avgolemono sauce

1 ½ cups of chick broth
1 egg separated
3 egg yolks
1 lemon juice
½ cup chicken broth
Salt and pepper

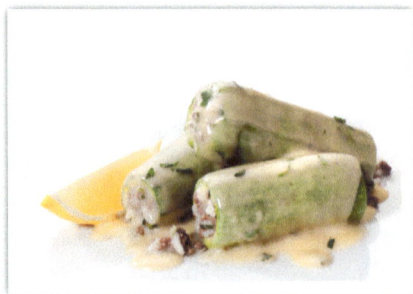

Guidance:

Bring broth to a boil and let it cool a little

In a bowl, whisk the egg whites until stiff, add egg yolks and continue beating until frothy.

Slowly whisk in the lemon juice followed by the hot liquid.

Whisk the mixture over medium heat until it thickens, about 5-10 minutes

Remove from heat and continue to stir for 1 minute.

Serve immediately with poached fish, boiled or steamed vegetables, dolmathes, stuffed zucchini and chicken dishes.

Guidance for stuffed zucchini:

Heat the oil in a pan.

Sauté the onions until tender

Add the garlic and sauté' but do not burn

Add the ground meat in the pan with the onions and cook until cooked

Drain any excess fat.

Add the garlic, parsley, dill, mint, lemon zest, rice, chicken stock and the inside of the zucchini that was removed before

Simmer for 20 minutes or until the rice is cooked.

Remove the pan from the heat and mix in the egg whites.

Stuff the zucchinis with the mixture

Place the stuffed zucchini in a pan.

Pour the chicken stock into the pan.

Cover and simmer for 20 minutes or until the zucchini is tender.

Plate the stuffed zucchini and use the remaining stock for the avgolemono sauce

Make the Avgolemono sauce and when you serve the finished stuffed zucchini you pour over 2-3 Tbsp. of the sauce. Savor it!

Stuffed zucchini flowers

The Zucchini flowers bloom in the spring. It is best to pick in the flowers in the morning when they are open so it will easier to stuff them.

Ingredients

50-60 zucchini flower blooms
2 cups of rice
1 chopped onion
1 diced fresh tomato
1.5 cups grated tomato
5 tbs. chopped parsley
4 tbs. chopped fresh mint
2 tbs. chopped basil
1/2 cup pine nuts
4 tbs. olive oil
3 cups of water
1.5 tsp ground pepper
Salt to taste
A pinch of cinnamon (optional)
2 tbs. olive oil per saucepan for coating

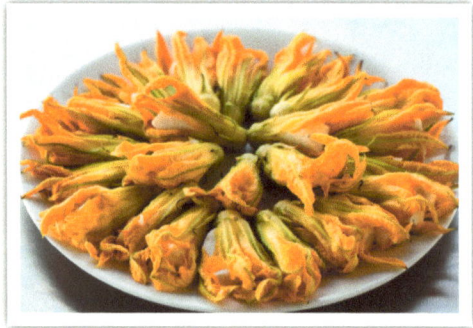

Instructions

1. Place the flowers in a large bowl of cold water and remove the stems. Drain the same.
2. In a separate bowl, mix the uncooked rice, onion, parsley, mint, basil, tomato, pine nuts, pepper, olive oil, salt and cinnamon.
3. Stuff each flower with a spoon with the mixture and fold over the ends of the petals. Repeat with all the zucchini flowers.
4. Sprinkle 2 tbs. olive oil at the bottom of a large saucepan
5. Arrange the stuffed flowers in a large saucepan side by side in a circular pattern. Do not pile the stuffed flowers on top of each other,

because the rice may result in being undercooked or overcooked. Make 2 pots if necessary

6. Place 1.5 cups of water in each saucepan, so that the water covers up to about half the height of the zucchini flowers.

7. Place a large ceramic plate covering the flowers on top of the saucepan. Cook the saucepan on the stovetop, on medium heat, for about 20-25 minutes, until most of the liquid has been absorbed. Enjoy!

Zucchini Fritters

Ingredients:

12-14 zucchinis
1 bunch (5-6) of scallions
    (or 1 large onion, diced)
1 clove of garlic, minced
1 large egg
2 Tbs. chopped fresh mint
2 Tbs. chopped fresh basil
1 Tbs. chopped fresh parsley
1 cup dried breadcrumbs
½ cup Graviera cheese, grated (or Asiago, Romano)
½ cup of Feta cheese, crumbled (optional)
½ tsp nutmeg
½ tsp. black pepper
Salt to taste
Oil for frying

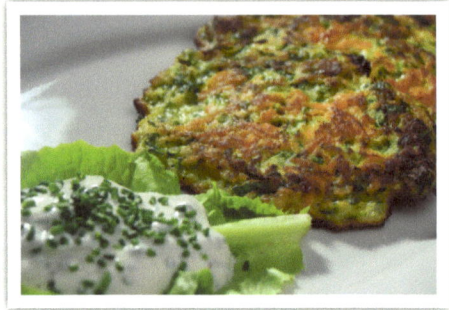

Instructions:

Rinse your zucchinis well and cut the ends off.

Shred the zucchinis and place them in a deep dish.

Sprinkle with some coarse sea salt, cover and let sit in the fridge for at least 3 hours

Squeeze out as much water as you can from the shredded zucchini. You can use your hands or a cheese cloth.

In a small skillet, add a couple of turns of olive oil, add your scallions and garlic into the skillet over medium heat.

Allow the fried scallions and garlic to cool before adding into the bowl with the zucchini.

Add the cooled scallion mixture, beaten egg, chopped herbs, nutmeg, breadcrumbs, crumbled Feta, grated Graviera, black pepper and mix with a spatula.

Mix the mixture, until you will be able to make patties with it. If the mixture is too dry, add a little olive oil and if the mixture is too wet, add some bread crumbs. Mix again.

Grab a small handful of the zucchini mixture in your hand and roll into a ball and then flatten into a patty. Make all the patties before frying.

Heat 1/2 inch of oil in a frying pan. Over medium heat, fry each patty until it's golden on both sides (approximately 3 minutes per side).

Transfer patties to a paper towel lined plate. Keep warm.

Best eaten warm on their own or with a cool dipping sauce like tzatziki or sour cream. Savor it!

Spinach Pie (Spanakopita)

This is "comfort food". This is truly my favorite. I can eat this for 3 days straight, breakfast, lunch and dinner. It's a flaky moist and salty delight. Can be an appetizer or a main dish.

Ingredients

1.5 lbs. chopped spinach, (you can substitute frozen, thawed and strained well)

~Can also substitute spinach with Chard (silver beet) but remove the stalks

½ cup olive oil

1 large onion, diced

2 bunches green onions, diced

½ cup parsley, chopped

½ cup fresh dill, chopped

¼ tsp. ground nutmeg

¼ tsp cinnamon

1 Tbsp. flour

Salt (1/2 tsp) and freshly ground black pepper to taste

1 cup feta cheese, crumbled

2 eggs, lightly beaten

½ cup ricotta cheese

¼ cup butter, melted

1/4 cup olive oil

1 lb. phyllo pastry sheets (Filo)

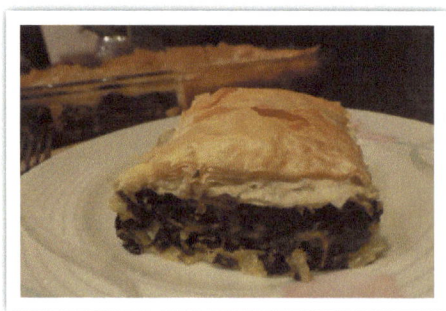

Instructions

Wash and drain the chopped spinach very well. If using frozen spinach, thaw completely and squeeze out excess water. Spinach should be dry.

Heat the olive oil in a deep sauté pan. Sauté the onions and green onions until tender. Add the spinach, parsley, dill, feta, ricotta, flour, eggs and cook for 5 to 10 minutes until the spinach is wilted and heated through. Add the nutmeg, cinnamon and season with salt and pepper. Mix until combined. At this point you should taste it to make sure it is slated to your liking.

If using frozen spinach, you will want to cook until excess moisture evaporates. Spinach mixture should be on the dry side.

Remove from heat, and set the spinach aside to cool.

Combine the melted butter with the olive oil in a bowl. Using a pastry brush, lightly grease one glass 9 x 12 rectangular pan.

Preparing the Pita

The plan: You will place 8 sheets of filo on the bottom of the pan, the spinach mixture in the middle and another 10 layers of filo on top.

Here is what to do:

Carefully remove the Phyllo roll from the plastic sleeve. Most packages come in 12 x 18-inch sheets when opened fully. Using a scissor or sharp knife, cut the sheets in half to make two stacks of 9x12 inch sheets. To prevent drying, cover one stack with wax paper and a damp paper towel while working with the other.

Layer about 8 sheets on the bottom of the pan by brushing each sheet with the butter/olive oil mixture. Add half of the spinach mixture in an even layer and press with a spatula to flatten. The filo will cover the inside side of the pan and you will fold it over.

Layer another 10 sheets on top of the spinach mixture making sure to brush well each sheet with butter/olive oil mixture.

Before baking, score the top layer of phyllo (making sure not to puncture filling layer) to enable easier cutting of pieces later. You can place the pan in the freezer to harden the top layers and then use a serrated knife.

Bake in a preheated 350-degree oven until the pita turns a deep golden brown for about 45 minutes, but keep watching it, you do not want to burn the filo.

~Eat a piece of spanakopita in my honor!

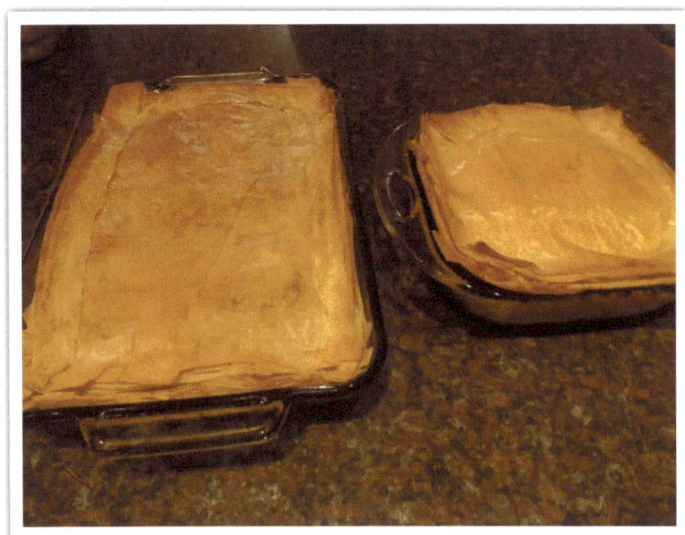

Peas and dill (Arakas)

4 Tbsp. extra-virgin olive oil

1 tsp of butter

1 medium yellow onion, peeled
and finely chopped

4-6 scallions, chopped

1 clove garlic, peeled and minced

4 cups shelled fresh or frozen peas

1/2 cup finely chopped dill

Salt and freshly ground black pepper

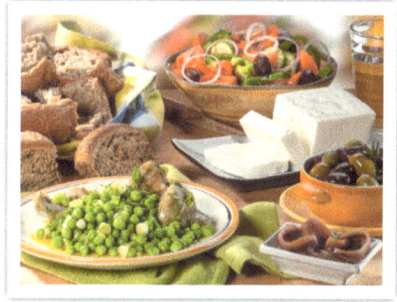

Variant:

(Arakas Kokistos) add tomato paste and oregano to the exact same recipe for a different taste

Instructions:

1. Heat oil and butter in a large deep pot over low heat. Add onions and garlic and keep stirring until onions become translucent, but not brown or burned. Stay on top of it and keep stirring

2. Add and stir in peas, dill and scallions. Add 1 cup of water just to cover, stirring occasionally, for 30 minutes. Keep the pot covered when you are not stirring.

3. Season with salt and pepper, and cook covered, while stirring every 20-30 minutes.

4. When the water has evaporated and peas "taste and look" cooked, turn off fire and serve.

5. Eat with feta cheese and a crusty bread (optional) on the side

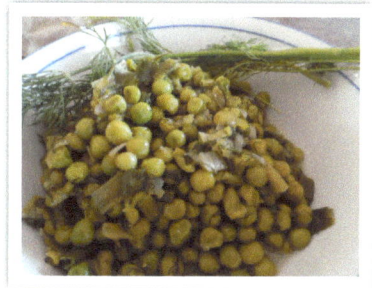

Stuffed grape leaves (dolmadakia)

This might be the hardest recipe in this publication, but the taste of fresh dolmadakia is nothing like the ones you buy in a can. This recipe can be eaten with a splash of lemon juice on top. A different version of this recipe is to add "avgolemono" sauce on top of warm dolmadakia. Both variants are excellent.

Either use vine leaves sold in jars or fresh. If you use the ones in jar, rinse the vine leaves, remove the stems and leave them in a sieve to drain. If using fresh vine leaves, wash them thoroughly, remove the stems and blanch them in boiling hot water. Remove the leaves with a slotted spoon and place them in a colander to cool down completely.

Ingredients

Vine leaves (approximately 40)
For the filling:
1/4 cup olive oil
1 cup scallions, finely chopped
3/4 cup medium grain rice
½ cup pine nuts
1/8 cup parsley, finely chopped
1/8 cup dill, finely chopped

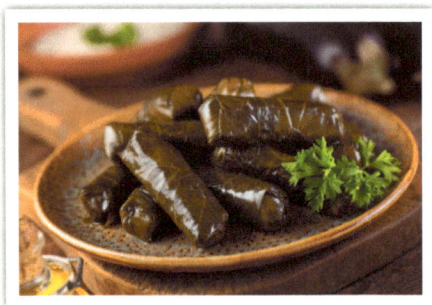

For the stock:

Juice of one lemon (about a ¼ cup)
1 cup dry white wine (optional)
3 cups vegetable or chicken stock
2 Tbsp. olive oil
Salt & pepper
Combine all of these ingredients in a separate bowl and place them on the side

Instructions

Rinse vine leaves before using. Handle with care, since they tear easily. Rinse the leaves in batches in a stockpot of warm water, drain. Remove stems and line up on your work surface, shiny side down.

In a large pan, sauté scallions in olive oil over medium heat, until lightly browned but not burned.

Add rice and pine nuts and sauté 2-3 minutes more until "married" together.

Add parsley and dill, wine, salt and pepper.

Lower heat, cover and simmer for 15 minutes, remove from heat to cool.

To fill the leaves:

Place 1 teaspoon of the rice mixture in the center of each leaf and fold the base up over the filling. Fold in each side and roll up into a secure cylinder. Be careful not to overfill the dolmades, as the rice will expand during cooking.

In a glass or cast-iron stock pot, layer the bottom of a large pot with some vine leaves.

Fold the lower section of the leaf over the filling towards the center; bring the two sides in toward the center and roll them up tightly. Place the stuffed vine leaves (folded side down) on the bottom of the pot in snug layers. Must be careful, not to leave any gaps between the dolmades to prevent them from cracking open while cooking.

Add the remaining stock mixture, and cover the rolled dolmadakia with a plate to keep them down and in place. Simmer gently over low heat for about an hour, or until tender.

Remove, drain and arrange on a platter to cool (or refrigerate until ready to use). Garnish with lemon wedges and dill sprigs. Best eaten the same day but can be stored in the refrigerator for up to one week. You can add an "Avgolemono" sauce before you serve them.

Egg and lemon chicken soup with rice (Avgolemono soupa)

This might sound like a strange recipe if you have never eaten it, but believe me it is a full-filling, thick, creamy (without flour), healthy and satisfying dish. The avgolemono sauce is made in a similar way. If you are a lemon lover, you will love this!

Ingredients

6 cups of water
½ cup of chicken base
1 cup of uncooked long-grain rice
3 eggs (room temperature)
¼ cup of fresh lemon juice
Sprinkle of lemon zest
2 tablespoons of cornstarch (optional)

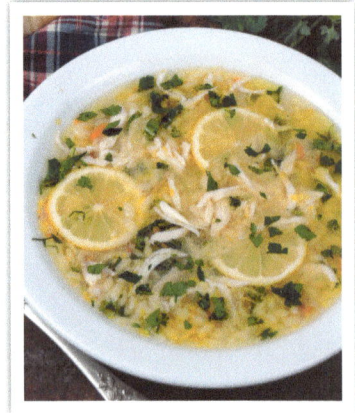

Instructions:

Eggs; separate the whites from yolks and keep them separate for now

Place water and chicken base in a pot

Stir until it boils

Add rice and bring to a boil again, add salt to taste and stir

Reduce heat, cover, and simmer for 15 -20 minutes.

Remove from heat. Let it cool down for 5 minutes.

In a large mixing bowl, beat egg whites until it becomes white and frothy

Add yolks,

Gradually beat in lemon juice and cornstarch into the mixing bowl

Add the lemon zest

Continue to beat the mixture until cornstarch dissolves.

Gradually add the COOLED (not hot) chicken base while continuing to beat the egg mixture.

Beat for a few more minutes; serve hot with some white pepper on top

Lentil soup (Fakes)

This was my children's favorite. They enjoy it while they were making fun of the "fakes" name to irritate me. It took me a while to get the joke. At least I gave them some healthy food while growing up. It's simple to make, and very healthy. Who needs meat every day?

Do not forget to use extra virgin olive oil, bay leaves, and a splash of red wine vinegar! Adding spinach can also be a delicious way to enjoy this dish in a separate way.

Ingredients:

1 lb. of lentils

1 medium onion, chopped

2-3 carrots medium sliced

2 cloves of garlic

1/2 cup of olive oil

8 oz. of chopped tomatoes (optional)

Half a bag of spinach (optional)

1-2 bay leaves

Salt and black pepper

2 tbs. Vinegar (balsamic, red wine or plain) to use right before eating

Instructions:

1. Clean and wash lentils and leave to soak in warm water for 2 hours
2. In a pot pour 6 cups water, lentils, chopped onion, carrots, (tomatoes), garlic and bay leaves.
3. Simmer 1 hour or so, lentil should be soft. Mixing often and gently
4. Add the oil, salt, pepper and (optional spinach)
5. Boil for another 15 minutes until well thickened.
6. Serve drizzled with a little vinegar feta and crusty bread on the side

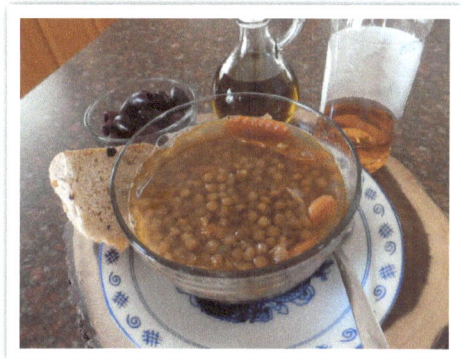

Santorini s Fava (Yellow split pea puree)

This is delectable "yellow heaven". If you feel weak, cold, depressed or just sick, this dish will "warm" you up. Fava peas, is an ancient food that has been found in Greece's archeological sites.

Ingredients:

500g (18 ounces) yellow split peas

3 red onions, roughly chopped

2 cloves of garlic, chopped

1 liter (3 cups) warm water

Juice of 2 lemons

1/3 of a cup olive oil

Dash of thyme

Salt and black pepper

Instructions:

Rinse the split peas with plenty of water 2-3 times.

Heat a large pot over medium-high heat; add 2-3 tsp. olive oil, the chopped onions, garlic and some fresh thyme and sauté.

As soon as the onions start to caramelize (but not burned) add the peas and blend for 1-2 min. Pour in the warm water (almost twice the quantity that is required to cover the peas) and the olive oil. Turn the heat down to medium and season well with salt and pepper. Simmer, and gently mix once in a while with the lid on for about 50-60 minutes, until the split peas are thick and mushy. While the split peas boil, some white foam will probably surface on the water. Remove the foam with a slotted spoon.

When done, pour in the lemon juice and transfer the mixture into a bowl. (Optional; press them with a fork to partially mush them). Mix, until the peas become smooth and creamy, like a chunky puree.

Top the fava with a drizzle (I like a lot) of olive oil, sprinkle lemon juice, 2-3 Kalamata olives, chopped green onions and serve. This plate is served warm. You will need a fork and good crusty high fiber bread to scoop up everything off the plate. I like this dish because it absorbs all the olive oil added to it.

Can you feel your toes curl up?

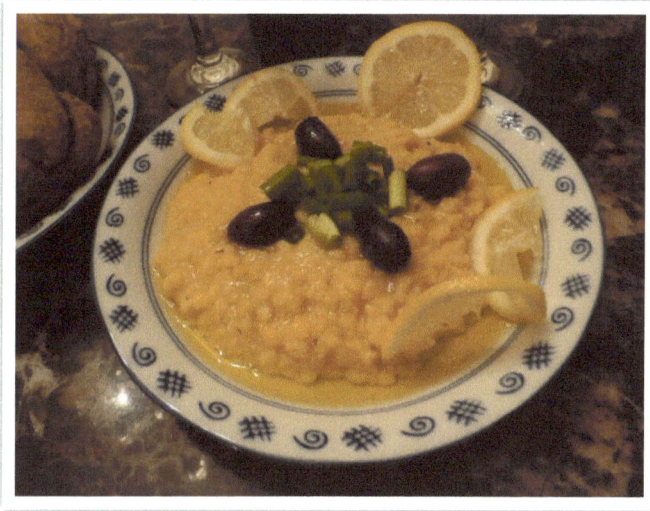

Fish soup (Kakavia)

The healthiest dish to calm your upset stomach after a long and hard day.

Ingredients

1/2 cup olive oil

2 large leeks, rinsed well & rough dice

3 carrots, peeled and chopped

2 stems of celery, chopped

3 large potatoes, diced

4 cloves of garlic, smashed

3 bay leaves

5-6 peppercorns

1-2 pinches of fresh thyme

1 pinch of saffron

1 cup dry white wine

2 red mullets (or 1 whole red snapper or Scorpion fish)

1 lb. clams

1lb. mussels

1 lb. shrimp, peeled & deveined

Save the shrimp shells and place them in a separate sachet

1 lb. white fish fillets (bass, haddock, halibut, whiting)

8-9 cups of water

salt and pepper to taste

crusty garlic bread

chopped fresh parsley

2-4 wedges of lemon

cheesecloth (place thyme, bay leaves, peppercorns, saffron and make a sachet inside the cloth, tie with a string)

Instructions:

In a large pot and over medium-high heat, add the olive oil

add the leeks, carrots and celery

Stir and sauté

Add the water

Add the sachet of herbs and another sachet of the shrimp shells

Lower to medium and cover for about 10 minutes.

Add the peeled potatoes; stir in for 1-2 minutes

Add the wine and water and bring to a boil

Cover, reduce to medium heat and simmer for another 30 minutes

Add salt and pepper to taste.

Add the whole fish (wrapped & tied in cheesecloth) and simmer for another 15 minutes. Carefully remove the fish and place it on the side, continue simmering the soup

Place the clams into the pot and bring back to a boil.

Once the soup is boiling, turn the heat off and add the mussels, shrimp and pieces of white fish and cooked red mullet meat. Cover and allow the residual heat of the soup to cook the seafood for about 10 minutes. Remove both sachets and discard.

Serve with lemons on the side and add salt and black pepper to taste

Beef soup with ribs and Bone Marrow

Bone marrow has a tremendous amount of nutritional value. There is calcium, selenium, phosphorus potassium and growth factors. Bone marrow is where the blood is formed, called hematopoiesis. In France, especially, they scoop the bone marrow and use it as a spread over their bread. In Greece, they often use it to make a good soup broth. This is an excellent soup for the winter. It is best to use organic beef long bones.

Ingredients:

1-1 ½ gallons Water

4 spareribs from beef

3-4 long bones with the marrow

1 lemon cut in half

2 pieces of celery

1 celery root (celeriac) in cubes

3 carrots sliced

2 yellow onions in quarters

1 potato peeled in cubes

Salt & pepper

½ cup of olive oil

2 bay leaves

½ beef bouillon (optional)

1 cinnamon stick (optional)

Instructions:

Place the meat and the bones in a large Pot

Add water, salt, pepper and half of the lemon

Simmer for 2 ½ hours with a closed lid until meat gets softened

Skim the froth from the broth to "clean" the appearance of the broth and let the broth cool down a little

Remove the meat and let it cool

Strain the broth and place in it another pot

Separate the meat from the ribs with your clean hands and add it to a new pot with the "clean" broth.

Add the potato (cinnamon stick, beef bouillon), carrot, celery, celeriac and olive oil to the new pot

Simmer for 30 minutes with the lid on.

The soup is ready to serve with lemon on the side

Giant Beans (Fasolada)

That is the poor man's pleasure. Enjoy it with a glass of wine (or more) and with your best friend. High in fiber, B vitamins, iron, protein, rich in phytonutrients and antioxidants!

Ingredients

18 oz. (500gr) dry giant white beans

8 cups of water

1 garlic clove, crushed

1-2 carrots, finely chopped

1 large red onion, finely chopped

3 stalks of celery, finely chopped

½ cup extra virgin olive oil

2 tbs. tomato puree

A pinch of paprika

A tbsp. of parsley

Salt and freshly ground pepper

Instructions:

Soak the beans in hot water for 2 hours. Not overnight!

Gently fry the onions, garlic, carrots and celery in olive oil for 10 minutes

Add tomato paste, salt and paprika

Cover and simmer for 10 minutes

Rinse the beans and add them to the rest of the mixture with the water

Cover and simmer for 2 hours or until beans are tender. Mixing occasionally.

Add parsley the last 30 minutes of cooking

Serve with a sprinkle of chopped parsley on top, some hard cheese on the side, and some crusty grainy bread.

It goes well with a glass of red wine!

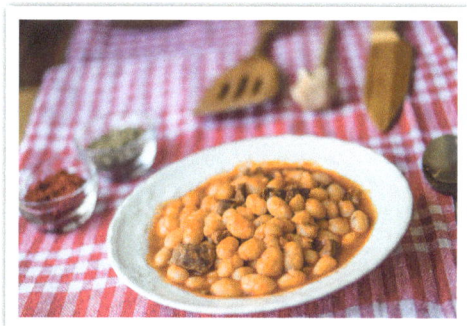

Yogurt and cucumber sauce (Tzatziki)

This is a side dish or a kind sauce-spread. Most people call it dip or sauce but it is a different concept. It is a cooling yogurt/cucumber sauce-spread that is placed on meats (as seen on Gyros) or on a crusty grainy bread and eaten as an appetizer. Please don't call it sauce! It's Tzatziki!

Ingredients

1 small cucumber

1 garlic clove, crushed

1 cup of Greek strained yogurt

2 teaspoons of lemon juice

1 teaspoon of dill (some substitute with mint)

Salt

Instructions:

Peel cucumber thinly and grate and place in strainer or cheesecloth to drain off the excess liquid. (Save the cucumber liquid for something else or to dilute the tzatziki if it becomes too thick)

Blend manually all ingredients together until you get a good thick consistency

Serve with fried fish or fried zucchini/eggplant slices

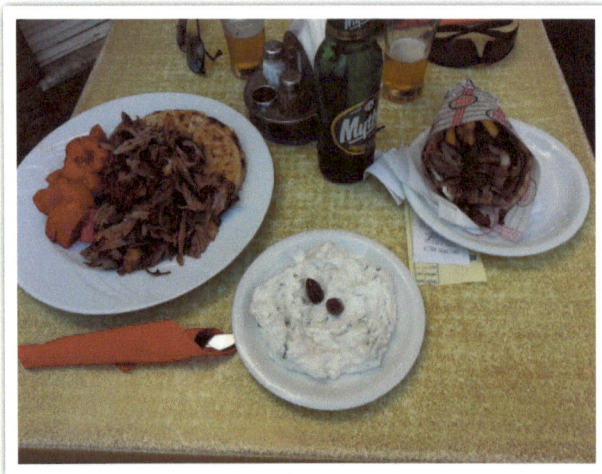

Skordalia (potato-garlic spread)

This is another "don't call it sauce" recipe, similar to tzatziki. If you are planning to kiss someone today do not eat this OR both of you must eat this. It is garlicky! If I have a sore throat or starting to get sick I eat this for few days and I am 200% better.

Ingredients:

1 medium potato

4 to 5 cloves garlic, peeled and minced

1 teaspoon kosher salt

1 cup olive oil

Juice of 1 lemon (about 1/4 cup)

1 large egg yolk

1/4 teaspoon ground black pepper

1/3 cup Kalamata olives, pitted and chopped

1/2 cup almonds or walnuts, toasted and ground (optional)

Mortar and pestle or a food processor.

Instructions:

Clean and peel the potatoes

Either boil or microwave the potatoes until cooked

Set aside until cool enough to handle.

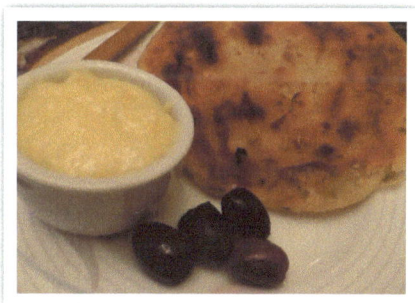

While potatoes cool, using a mortar and pestle to crush the garlic and salt together into a fine paste.

In a glass bowl (or food processor) add the cool potatoes and start mashing.

Slowly and gradually add the garlic paste, egg yolk, black pepper, olives, (almonds), lemon juice, and olive oil to the potatoes and mix well, until it has the consistency of mashed potatoes.

Adjust the consistency and taste with more olive oil, salt, and pepper, and serve.

It is best on a slice of hardy crusty bread or with a dry fish like Cod.

Baked fish

The easiest dish to make. Even a student can make it. This is an all protein meal to feed your muscles and provide phosphorus to your eyes. Simple and nutritious

Ingredients:

3-4 white fish filets (frozen is fine)

½ cup of olive oil

½ juice of a lemon

Dash of Paprika

Oregano

Salt

Instructions:

Place the fish in a glass baking pan

Add the olive oil over the fish fillet

Sprinkle the oregano, lemon juice over the fish

Sprinkle paprika over the fish filets

Bake for 20 minutes

The juice with the oil that comes in the pan can be sprinkled over your side dish (rice pilaf). Never waste the olive oil and lemon juice

Serve and savor!

Meat balls in sauce (souzoukakia)

Ingredients:

500g ground beef (1 lb.)

500g ground veal or pork (1 lb.)

4 cloves of garlic, crushed

2 eggs beaten

1 tsp of ground cumin (optional)

½ tsp of ground cinnamon

¼ tsp of ground clove

½ cup of white wine

2 cups of tomato sauce

1 cup of breadcrumbs

2 tsp of salt and freshly ground
   pepper

Olive oil for frying

Instructions:

Mix all the ingredients together except the tomato sauce and the oil

Moisten your hands with water and shape the mixture into sausage-like rolls about 8 cm (3 inches) long.

First fry the meatballs in a pan with oil and then

place the sausage-like rolls inside the tomato sauce and simmer them for 1 hr.

Souzoukakia can be served over spaghetti or on the side of a rice pilaf dish.

Eggplant & Beef (Moussaka)

Any publication on Greek food will not be complete unless we mention Moussaka.

Moussaka is the favorite dish of all the tourists that visit Greece. It is full of flavor, and a filling food.

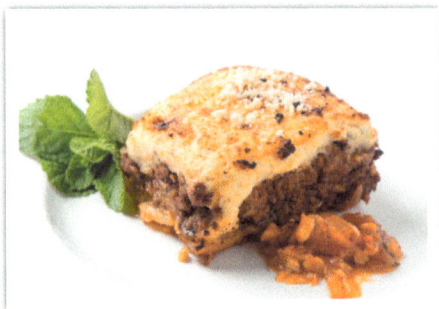

There are 3 separate parts and layers to make, then place them all together in a deep bake Pyrex dish which bakes in the oven. Since this dish is so rich, it is often enjoyed with a Greek salad on the side.

Plan:

First make the ground meat, then the sauce, and then the eggplant. Place the eggplants on the bottom on the cooking dish, the ground meat on top and then the béchamel sauce on top. Then you bake the dish.

Finally, you can savor your food!

Step 1: Make the Ground Beef

Ingredients

1 lb. ground beef

1 medium onion, diced

3 Tbsp. olive oil

2 cloves garlic, finely minced

¼ cup red wine

¼ cup chopped fresh parsley

½ tsp. ground cinnamon

2 bay leaves

¼ ground cloves

A pinch of allspice

Salt and ground black pepper to taste

2 oz. (55g) can tomato paste

½ teaspoon sugar

1 cup water

Place olive oil in the pan at medium heat

Place the chopped onion in the oiled pan and sauté until translucent

Add the ground beef, garlic, cinnamon, clove, allspice, parsley, salt and pepper

Once the ground meat is cooked, add the water, tomato paste, bay leaves and sugar

Bring to a boil, and then simmer with the pan lid on until the water evaporates (about 30-40 min). Make sure you keep mixing it every 5 minutes.

Taste it, to make sure it's done right

Grease a 9 x 9-inch baking pan, although you could use a 13 x 9 pan as well, using a smaller pan, will result in a thicker casserole.

Step 2: Make the eggplant

Ingredients:

2 medium eggplants   salt and pepper
1 cup of olive oil

Peel the eggplant, then slice into 1/4-inch thick slices (or a little thicker won't hurt).

Brush a cookie sheet with olive oil. This part of the eggplant preparation can be used in other dishes for variety; such as a spaghetti toping or over rice.

Coat each side of sliced eggplant with olive oil then season slices with salt and fresh ground pepper.

Place the eggplant slices on cookie sheet and broil until brown

Turn and broil the other side, brushing all eggplant slices with extra olive oil if needed.

In the bottom of the prepared baking dish arrange half of the eggplant slices.

Step 3: Make the Béchamel sauce:

Ingredients:

5 tablespoons butter

1/2 teaspoon salt

1/2 teaspoon fresh ground black
   pepper

2 tablespoons flour

1 cup half-and-half cream

1 egg

1/2 -1 cup grated parmesan
   cheese

Melt the butter in a saucepan, whisk in flour, 1/2 tsp salt and pepper to taste; gradually stir in half and half (or milk)

Cook and stir over medium heat until thick and bubbly.

In a small bowl, beat egg; stir in some of the warm sauce into the beaten eggs,

Then add the beaten eggs to sauce mixture

Mix well

Add in Parmesan cheese, and stir again

It's ready when it's thickened. Remove from the heat but keep it warm until you are ready to pour it over the top layer.

Step 4: Place all the steps together

Place the eggplant slices on the bottom of the cooking dish, layer the ground meat on top of eggplant slices and spread to cover them.

Place the béchamel sauce on top of the ground meat and spread to cover it.

Bake in a preheated 350-degree F oven for 45 minutes.

Braised beef and onion stew (Stifado)

This is a delicious beef stew recipe, that is very tender and melts in your mouth. The taste is slightly sweet and hardy.

Ingredients:

3 lbs. good-quality stewing beef, cut into portions

2 lbs. baby shallot onions, peeled

¼ cup of olive oil

1 cup of red wine

1/3 cup of cognac

3 Tbs. red wine vinegar

1 large ripe chopped tomato

1 tsp tomato purée

1 bay leaf

3-4 allspice berries

1 pinch of nutmeg

1 pinch of cinnamon

salt and pepper

½ cup of boiled water

Heat the olive oil in a saucepan, add the meat and sauté, until browned on all sides. When done, remove the meat, place on a plate, cover and set aside.

Clean the baby shallot onions and add in the same oil used to brown the meat and sauté on low heat until the onions have softened (about 10 minutes).

In a crock pot, add all ingredients, including the meat, onions and hot water, cook on low heat for 4 hours. While the beef stifado is simmering, check to see that it remains moist, if it starts to dry out, add water, because it should remain moist.

This dish is served with rice pilaf on the side. Enjoy!

Stuffed cabbage leaves (lahano dolmathes)

Ingredients:

1 medium cabbage (about 24 leaves)

1 lb. beef/pork mince (or mixed)

200 ml 1/3 cup of short-grain white rice (uncooked)

2 spring onions, chopped

1 tomato peeled and chopped

1 onion, chopped

2 Tbs. of parsley, finely chopped

1 tsp. of dill or mint, finely chopped

1/8 tsp. ground cinnamon

2 Tbs. olive oil

Salt & pepper

2 eggs

Juice of 1 lemon

1 Tbs. of butter

1 tbsp. corn flour (optional)

To make the stuffing:

Gently fry the onions in olive oil until soft.

Mix in the meat with uncooked rice, tomato, parsley, dill or mint, cinnamon, salt & pepper

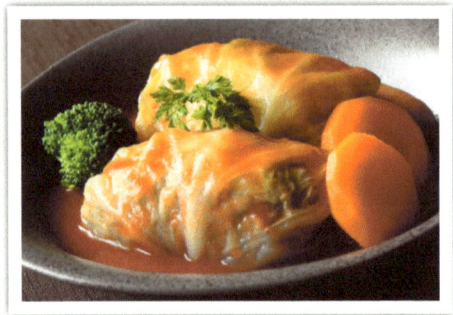

Instructions:

1. Blanching the cabbage leaves: Put the cabbage in a pot with about 2/3 water full, boil on medium heat until the leaves are tender and begin to open.

2. Remove and drain the cabbage leaves when soft but firm.

3. Combine the minced meat mixture in a large bowl. Add a splash of olive oil and season to taste with salt and pepper.

4. Lay a cabbage leaf on the counter surface in front of you. Place about a tbsp. of the mince meat mixture at the base of the leaf. Wrap once and then fold inwards, and fold the sides toward the center, to form a small parcel. Proceed and roll up all of your cabbage rolls.

5. In a big pot, arrange a couple of cabbage leaves to cover the base of the pot. Place your cabbage rolls on top, making sure to pack the rolls close together with the seam side down. If necessary, start a new layer.

6. Add water over your rolls, a splash of oil, butter and season to taste with salt and pepper.

7. Cover your rolls with a dinner plate turned upside down, to help them retain their shape while cooking. Replace the lid on the pot. Some people use a pressure cooker; in that case, there is no need for the plate over the rolls.

8. Simmer gently for 1 ½ hours depending on the level of water you placed in

9. When cooked, drain off the stock carefully in a separate container for possible use later, and then transfer the cabbage rolls into a small saucepan.

10. Prepare the egg-lemon sauce by whisking 2 eggs together with the juice of 1 lemon. If you prefer a thicker sauce, whisk the tbsp. of corn flour into the mixture.

11. While whisking the egg-lemon mixture, add a few spoonsful of the liquid from the pot containing the cabbage rolls. This will prevent the eggs from coagulating. Pour this mixture over the rolls. Grab the pot by its handles and shake it gently to ensure that the sauce permeates through the rolls.

12. Enjoy!

Chicken a la Ferrugia

This recipe was given from an old friend, Michelle Epifano-Gidosh, and it is an old family recipe. Una vecchia ricetta di famiglia!

Ingredients

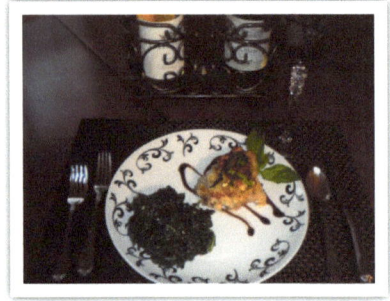

6-8 pieces of chicken parts (keep skin and bones intact)
(works best with chicken thighs)
6-8 cloves of fresh garlic, chopped
4-5 Fresh basil leaves, chopped
1 tablespoon of dry Italian seasonings
(oregano, basil, rosemary and thyme)
One small can of tomato sauce thinned with water
(two-parts sauce, one-part water).

Instructions:

Rinse chicken parts and arrange in a large roasting pan

Sprinkle fresh garlic, dry Italian seasonings, salt and pepper, over and under the skin of each chicken part. Spoon tomato sauce & water mixture over the top of each chicken part

Bake for 40-50 minutes at 400° or until chicken is thoroughly cooked

Garnish with fresh basil, and serve with your favorite vegetable as a side dish, and a nice Italian wine

La vita è bella!

Spinach with rice (as a side dish with the chicken recipe above)

Ingredients

1/3 cup of olive oil

2 green onions chopped

2 lbs. of fresh spinach

-(rinsed and stemmed)

1 tsp of dill chopped

1 tsp of Italian parsley

1 cup of tomato sauce

2 cups of water (or chicken broth)

½ cup of uncooked white rice

Salt and pepper to taste

Instructions:

Heat olive oil in a large skillet over medium-high heat. Sauté onions in the oil until soft. Add spinach, parsley and dill and cook while stirring for about 1-2 minutes, then pour in the tomato sauce and water. Bring to a boil and add salt and pepper. Stir in rice, reduce heat to low, and simmer uncovered for 20 to 25 minutes, or until rice is tender. Add more water if necessary. Enjoy

Blanquette de Veau

The French are famous for love, wine and Blanquette de Veau, the French veal ragout. This dish is important, and has become a classic of bourgeois cookery!

Ingredients:

1 ½ cups of cleaned pearl onions

4 ½ lbs. (2 kg) veal shoulder, boned, trimmed, cut into cubes

8 cups of chicken broth

3 fresh thyme sprigs

2 bay leaves

5 tablespoons butter

1 ½ lbs. (500g) celeriac (celery root), peeled, cut into 1 ½ inch (4 cm) pieces

4 large carrots, peeled, cut into 1 ½ inch (4 cm) lengths

3 medium turnips, peeled, each cut into 6 pieces

8 ounces button mushrooms

6 ounces green beans, trimmed and cleaned

3 tablespoons all-purpose flour

1/2 cup heavy cream

1/2 tablespoon fresh lemon juice

1/2 bunch chopped fresh chives

Instructions:

Bring large pot of salted water to boil.

Add pearl onions and cook 1 minute.

Using slotted spoon, remove onions from pot. Trim ends and peel.

Add veal to pot and cook 4 minutes.

Drain veal and rinse with cold water.

Rinse pot and return veal to pot.

Add 10 cups chicken broth and bring to boil.

Reduce heat and simmer 30 minutes.

Add thyme and bay leaves and simmer until veal is tender, stirring occasionally, about 30 minutes longer.

Melt 2 tablespoons butter in separate heavy large pot over medium heat.

Add pearl onions, celery root, carrots, turnips, mushrooms and 1 cup chicken stock. Cover and cook until vegetables are tender and almost all liquid has evaporated, about 15 minutes.

Add string beans and cook until just tender, about 2 minutes.

Drain veal, save 2 cups liquid and mix veal into vegetables.

Make to "Roux": Mix in 3 tablespoons flour into the melted butter from before, over medium heat. Cook until butter mixture turns golden brown, about 2 minutes, stirring constantly. Whisk in 2 cups of the saved cooking liquid.

Cook until thickened, about 5 minutes, stirring frequently.

Stir in heavy cream.

Season sauce to taste with fresh lemon juice, salt and pepper.

Pour cream sauce over cooked veal and vegetables.

Garnish with fresh chives and serve immediately. Red Bordeaux is suggested with this dish.

Bon appetit mon ami!

String Beans in tomato sauce

1 Kg (2 lbs.) cleaned string beans
2 potatoes
1 yellow onion chopped
3 cloves of garlic
½ Kg (1 lb.) fresh tomatoes
    chopped

1 Tsp tomato paste
½ cup parsley chopped
¼ cup dill chopped
1 cup of olive oil
1 cup of water
Salt and pepper

Instructions:

In a heated deep pot add ½ cup of olive oil

Gently fry onion and garlic in oil until onions are transparent not burned!

Add the string beans and keep stirring for 5 minutes

Add the potatoes, dill, parsley, tomatoes and stir for 5 minutes

Add the water, tomato paste, salt and pepper

Bring to a boil and then reduce the heat and simmer for 40-45 minutes

Keep stirring until ready

Serve with feta and bread on the side

Braised Artichokes

12 globe artichoke hearts

½ cup of chopped spring onions

500 g (1 lb.) baby carrots, scraped

12 button onions, peeled

12 small potatoes

Juice of 1 lemon

1 cup of olive oil

Water or chicken stock

Salt & pepper

Fresh dill or parsley, chopped

4 tsp. corn-flour

Instructions:

Wash artichokes well and cut off stems close to base

Have ready a bowl of cold water with the juice of 1 lemon and some lemon slices added

Line a wide based sauce pan with spring onions

Arrange carrots, whole onions, potatoes and artichoke hearts on top of spring onions

Add lemon juice, olive oil and enough water or chicken stock to barely cover

Season with salt and pepper to taste and sprinkle 1 tsp. of dill or parsley over the vegetables

Cover and simmer for 30 minutes or until vegetables are tender

Remove large vegetables to a heated platter with a slotted spoon, arrange them attractively.

Keep warm

Mix corn-flour into the pan with the left-over juice of the vegetables.

Mix into a paste with a little cold water and thicken liquid in pan.

Let it boil gently for 2 minutes

Pour sauce over vegetables and garnish with additional chopped herbs

Braised okra (Mbamies Yahni)

Ingredients:

1.5 lb. (750 g) fresh okra
½ cup of plain vinegar
1 large onion, sliced
2 garlic cloves crushed
½ cup of oil
2 cups chopped, peeled tomatoes
1 Tbs. chopped parsley
½ teaspoon sugar
Salt & Pepper

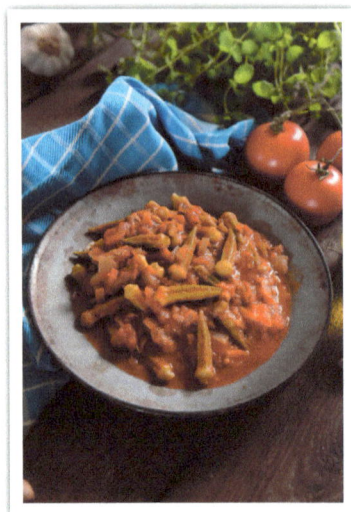

Instructions:

Wash okra and trim stalks but do not remove cone shaped tops

Place in a bowl, pour vinegar over and soak them for 30 minutes

Drain, rinse well and dry with paper towels

Gently fry onion and garlic in oil until onions are transparent not burned!

Add the dried okra and toss gently in pan, sauté them until slightly browned

Add remaining ingredients, salt and pepper to taste

Cover and simmer gently for 30-40 minutes until tender, depending on size of okra.

Sprinkle with additional chopped parsley and serve hot or cold as a side dish or as a main dish with some cheese and a slice whole grain bread.

Tip: okra can be substituted for string beans, sliced zucchini, sliced eggplant. Just do not soak them in vinegar.

Lamb Stew

This is Dr. Theo's original recipe. It comes out so soft and juicy. Since I live in beautiful Arizona and like to cook outside, my neighbors are getting very jealous with the aromas of my creations, especially this one.

Ingredients:

1 Boneless leg of lamb

5-8 red potatoes

4 bay leaves

10 whole cloves

1 cinnamon stick

1 Tbs. fennel seeds

½ cup of sangria

2 Tbs. of garlic powder

Salt and pepper to taste

Crock pot

Instructions:

Wash and cut up the leg of lamb into 3 parts.

Place the meat inside the crock pot

Place the clean and peeled potatoes with the meat

Sprinkle and massage the garlic powder and salt all over the meat.

Place the whole cloves inside the crevasses of the meat. Take a pointy knife and make jabs on the meat and stick the cloves inside the meat.

Strategically place the bay leaves under and around the meat

Place the cinnamon stick under the meat

Massage the fennel seeds all over the meat

Drench the meat with the wine

Start the crock pot at high for 1 hour and then at low for 4 more hours

Remove the meat and place it in the oven for 10-15 minutes if you like a drier meat (optional)

Skordalia and a tomato salad compliment well this dish.

Eggplant stew

Ingredients:

1 kilo (2 lbs.) Japanese eggplant

2/3 cup olive oil

2 cups onions, thinly sliced

3-4 garlic cloves, peeled and
   sliced thin

2 cups tomatoes, peeled and
   sliced

1/2 cup water

1 teaspoon oregano

½ cup of chopped parsley

1 teaspoon sugar

Instructions:

Preheat oven to 350C (180F).

Cut the stalks off the eggplant and rinse them well.

Make 2 evenly deep incisions lengthwise in each eggplant and soak in a bowl of salted water for 1 hour to remove the bitterness

Drain and dry well, squeezing eggplant gently to remove moisture.

Slice the eggplant on one side only, making them able to be opened up like a book, using care without breaking them.

Add a little bit of oil in a frying pan and shallow fry the eggplant on all sides.

Remove the eggplant from the frying pan and place into an oven-safe dish (side by side), and season them with salt, pepper and oregano.

Sauté the onions and garlic in the frying pan, slightly golden.

Add the chopped tomatoes and parsley along with one cup of water.

Stir and add salt and pepper to taste.

Sprinkle a touch of sugar into the mixture and stir well, cover and cook for 15 minutes.

Carefully stuff the eggplant with the mixture, using a small spoon while making sure not to break them.

Place the oven-safe saucepan into the preheated oven.

Bake for 40 minutes, sprinkling water once or twice on them during this period

Remove and savor!

Beetroot salad

This is an excellent and refreshing dish for the summer.
The taste is enhanced with Skordalia on the side.

Ingredients:

2 tsp ground cloves

1 tsp minced garlic

2 tbsp. finely chopped fresh
mint

1 tbsp. finely chopped fresh
parsley

1 ½ tsp ground coriander seeds

1 tsp sea salt

½ tsp fresh ground black pepper

3 tsp good quality Greek
olive oil

2 tsp good quality red wine
vinegar

Instructions:

Boil the beets ahead of time in water, for approximately 1 hour until easily pierced with a fork

Drain, and once cooled, peel and chop the beets

Add chopped beets and the remaining ingredients into a bowl, and gently stir to combine well. Take your time, and do not rush this step, the ingredients need time to "marry."

Serve as a side dish or a light snack. This dish goes well with skordalia on the side.

Dandelion Greens / Radikia

Ingredients:

2-3 lbs. of Dandelion leaves
   (greens)

Salt

6-8 cups of water to boil

1 cup of olive oil

½ lemon

Instructions:

Cut and chop the dandelion leaves. The stems are sweet so keep them on

Wash well and let them soak in cold water for 2-3 minutes to freshen up. Drain

Boil water with enough salt to remove the bitterness of the greens

Add the dandelion leaves into the boiling water

Make sure you push them down with a wooden spoon to keep them submerged

Bring to a boil for 4-5 min (if fresh) or 10 min if store bought.

Scoop out the greens with tongs and let them drain

Place the greens into a deep dish and dress them with a heavy dose of your finest olive oil, and a little bit of lemon juice to your taste.

This dish can be eaten with some feta cheese on the side and a Kouloura from Crete.

Greek Salad

Greek salad also known as "village salad" is simple to make and it's perfect for the summer with a beer.

Ingredients:

2-3 Organic tomatoes

2 chucks of Feta cheese

6 Kalamata olives

1 red onion in slices

½ Tbs. dried oregano

½ cucumber in round slices

½ green bell pepper

Top quality of olive oil

1 Tbs. balsamic vinegar

Sea salt

Freshly ground pepper to taste

Instructions:

Cut the tomatoes into wedges

Cut the onions into slices and into quarters

Peel and cut the cucumbers into slices

Cut the bell pepper into slices and quarters

Mix all the ingredients together, and top the salad with olive oil and oregano

Mix well with a spoon before eating

For this dish you need a good crusty whole wheat bread to soak up and eat all the olive oil.

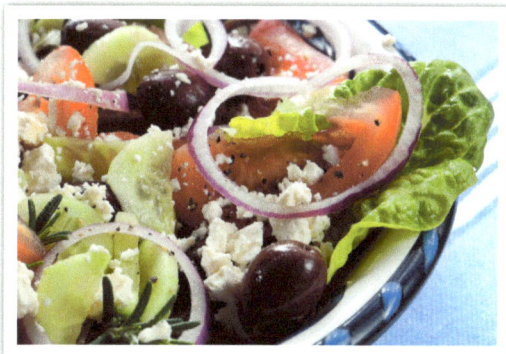

Baklava

This is a nutritious sweet dish that is enjoyed with a nice cup of strong coffee, while relaxing at an outdoor coffee shop with a friend. "Greeks do not eat walnuts they eat Baklava"

Greek Baklava is made with a lot of walnuts and real honey. The filling is thick not just a spread. A good baklava has quality ingredients so don't complain if you pay $5.00 for a good piece of homemade Baklava. Other cultures use pistachios or almonds in their Baklava

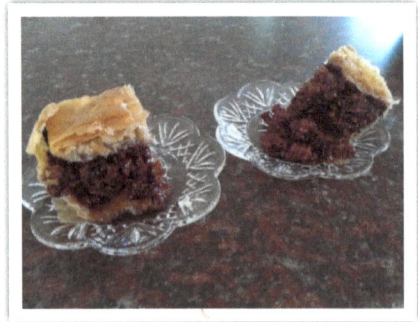

Ingredients:

1 1/2 pounds walnuts, chopped
1 cup of honey
1/2 teaspoon cinnamon
1/8 teaspoon ground cloves
Nutmeg (optional)
Zest of 1 lemon

Zest of half orange
1 shot of Amaretto liqueur
40 sheets Filo Dough (9 x 14), thawed
1 cup melted butter, olive oil, or cooking spray

Instructions:

In a medium bowl, combine walnuts, honey, cinnamon, cloves, nutmeg, amaretto, and finely chopped orange and lemon zest. This is the walnut filling that will go in between the filo layers.
Lightly spray a 9" x 13" baking pan with cooking spray.
Place 20 sheets of filo on the bottom of the pan, brushing each sheet with melted butter
Cover with 1/2 of the walnut mixture.

Layer 5 more filo sheets on top, brushing each sheet with butter (or lightly spraying with cooking spray.)

Spread the remaining half of the walnut mixture over the filo

Cover with another 15 sheets of filo, brushing each sheet with butter or olive oil (or lightly spray with cooking spray)

With a sharp knife, score the top layer of filo into 1 ½" diamonds or squares. Brush the top with butter so it bakes golden brown.

Bake in preheated 350°F oven for 45 minutes to 1 hour or until golden brown.

Cool slightly and pour cool warm syrup evenly over baklava.

Cool completely, cut and serve.

Syrup for baklava I must admit that this is the hardest thing to make. The syrup must be thick once you are done with it.

Ingredients:

2.5 cups granulated sugar

1 cup honey

2 cups water

1 lemon peel

1 cinnamon stick

3 cloves

1 tablespoon of lemon juice

Instructions: Bring all ingredients to a boil. Simmer for 10 minutes. Remove any foam from the top. Strain and cool slightly. Pour warm syrup over baklava. Cool completely, cut and serve.

Greek Coffee

It is like an espresso but it has sediment which should not be consumed. It can include sugar but not milk.

Ingredients:

1 tablespoon of Greek coffee (it is not the same as any other coffee)

Sugar (optional)

1 briki

Demitasse cups

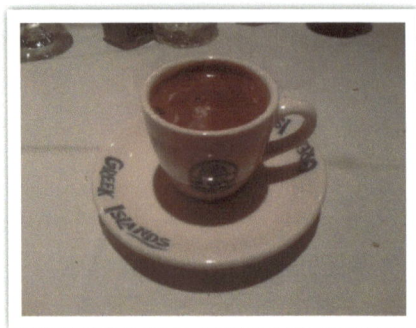

Instructions:

Using one of your demitasse cups as a 2-ounce measure, fill the briki with as many cups of cold water as cups of coffee you want to make. Add 1 heaping teaspoon of coffee grounds for each 2-ounce cup of coffee. Add granulated sugar, if desired

In the Briki you add:

2 oz. of water

1 heaping tsp Greek coffee

1 tsp of sugar (this is medium sweet, if you like sweeter you can add more)

Mix well and start heating up the Briki over the stove.

Do not continue to stir.

Stay and watch the coffee

Once the coffee starts bubbling up and makes a frothy top remove it from the heat.

Tap the briki 2 times on the counter and pour inside the cup

Enjoy!

Glossary

Physician: A licensed professional that diagnoses, treats and practices medicine. A physician can practice general medicine or any one of the numerous medical specialties.

Doctor: Doctor comes from the latin "Docere" and the Greek "Didactor" which means "to teach". A doctor is the professional that has achieved the highest level of education in their field of study. A physician is most likely a Doctor but not all Doctors are physicians.

Medicine: is the profession that deals with the diagnosis and treatment of humans or animals. There are numerous medical specialties that support and complement the practice of medicine.

Naturopathic Medicine: A field of scientific and evidence based medicine that has an integrative approach in the diagnosis and treatment of diseases in humans. The philosophic approach is to treat the cause of the disease by treating the whole person using the least harmful ways and educating the patient. This type of medicine has gained acceptance and popularity by licensing the profession in 20 states, so far, in the United States of America. This type of medicine is a unique and American grown medical specialty that has "blended" the scientific and traditional approaches of several types of medical philosophies. It has an individualized approach that emphasizes prevention, wellness and patient accountability. It is an effective type of medicine for chronic diseases and wellness.

Allopathic Medicine: a field of medicine that emphasizes the emergency approach of life threatening situations by using pharmaceutical medications and surgery. The philosophic approach is based on public health; alleviate suffering and not so much on individual treatment. Allopathic medicine uses pharmaceutical medications that are often "toxic" and have many side effects. It is an effective type of medicine for emergency situations and palliative care.

Naturopathic Physician: Licensed physicians in their respective state that practice medicine using integrative and personalized approaches. Depending on the state licensure, naturopathic physicians can prescribe medications and perform minor surgery in addition to using botanical, physical, nutritional and oriental medical approaches.

Chronic Diseases: "A disease that persists for a long time. A chronic disease is one lasting 3 months or more, by the definition of the U.S. National Center for Health Statistics. Chronic diseases generally cannot be prevented by vaccines or cured by medication, nor do they just disappear. 88% of Americans over 65 years of age have at least one chronic health condition (as of 1998). Health damaging behaviors, particularly tobacco use, lack of physical activity, and poor eating habits are major contributors to the leading chronic diseases". (Medicinenet. com) Heart disease, stroke, cancer, type 2 diabetes, obesity, and arthritis are among the most common chronic diseases.

ASCP: The American Association of Clinical Pathology is the organization that provides certification and education for pathologists and laboratory professionals.

Diseases of affluence: certain types of diseases and health conditions that are the result of increased wealth in a society often seen in "western countries". Diseases of affluence are caused by over-consumption of food and physical inactivity. Those diseases are in contrast to "the diseases of poverty". These diseases are linked with obesity, cardiovascular disease, high blood pressure, diabetes, metabolic syndrome, osteoporosis, colorectal cancer, acne, gout, depression, and diseases related to vitamin and mineral deficiencies.

Diet: is the specific intake of nutrition for health or weight-management reasons. Diet is a specific consumption of nutrients for a specific health concern.

Nutrition: is the type of nourishment an individual or organism consumes. Nutrition is the science of food consumption of nutrients and other substances in food as it relates to health and disease.

Mediterranean: "Middle earth" is the region that is around the Mediterranean Sea that includes Greece, Italy, France and Spain. North Africa and eastern Middle East are not usually included in that region even though they are proximal to the area.

Mediterranean Diet: The nutritional recommendations that provides health benefits, originally inspired by the dietary patterns of Greece, Italy, France and Spain. It is mostly the traditional Greek diet, that originated in the island of Crete.

Polyphenols: Polyphenols are phytochemicals, compounds found in natural plant food sources that have antioxidant properties. Antioxidants protect the body of free radicals that damage the cells.

www.ingramcontent.com/pod-product-compliance
Lightning Source LLC
Chambersburg PA
CBHW040929030426
42334CB00002B/12